Aphasia Recovery Connection's

Guide to Living with Aphasia

by
Carol Dow-Richards, ARC Director
and
Amanda P. Anderson M.S., CCC-SLP

With Christine Huggins and David Dow

A Message from the ARC Co-Founders

(cover photo)

We had strokes and have aphasia. We know how lonely the road to recovery can be. It is frightening, embarrassing at times, and overwhelming.

We hope this book will help you on your road to recovery. Recovery is often a long and slow process.

At times, it may feel like you aren't making any gains but gains come in many ways. Gains in speech, reading, writing, processing and understanding language. Gains in confidence. Gains in motivation. Gains in understanding aphasia. Gains in adapting to an invisible disability.

You can start this book at any chapter—feel free to jump in. *Share with family and friends because APHASIA RECOVERY is a team effort. Communication is a two-way street, and with your new challenges, it is a good idea to enlist some help from others.*

We hope you'll join us on ARC, our Facebook site. You could also take part in a cruise or join us at one of our ARC Aphasia Boot Camps. Keep trying—it is a lot of work! We know; We have travelled this road as well.

You are not alone,
Christine Huggins
David Dow

Table of Contents

Aphasia Recovery Connection
Leadership Team
Founders

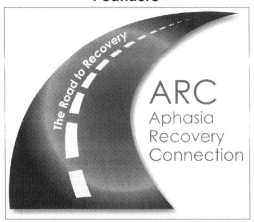

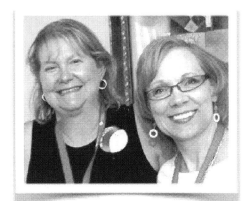

**Kim Huggins
Carol Dow-Richards**

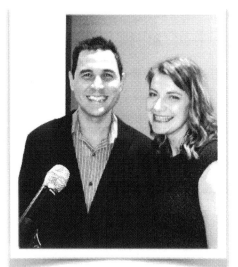

**David Dow
Christine Huggins
Stroke Survivors with Aphasia**

A Thank You

From the ARC Leadership Team

On behalf of people dealing with aphasia, we want to thank Amanda Anderson for her dedication to this project as we aim to help families navigate the road to recovery. Having the voice of an aphasia clinician and author has given the book a unified voice for all the experts: clinicians, patients, and families. Her generous donation of countless hours writing, editing, designing, and producing the content are so appreciated. Her commitment to ARC and to people with aphasia will make a difference today and for years to come.

Thank you to our editors Jean-François Brissette, Melinda Bell, and Linda Lauria who put in not only their time and energy, but their true compassion into helping families dealing with aphasia. Thank you to the graphic design firm company Annamedia, who has shown creativity and insight during the designing process for our cover, logo, and other design needs.

Thank you to our families who supported our time commitment to get this book into the hands of those who will benefit from it.

The ARC leadership team has selflessly donated their time over the last two years to make the dream of ARC as a non-profit organization a reality. We can't do it alone. In order to grow, we need the help of others to support our mission. If you would like to make a difference and help ARC grow, please consider ARC in your financial giving or bequest planning. Because we are a non-profit all donations are tax deductible. We are a young and driven non-profit that can only grow with the support of time, energy, and financial resources.

We are here with you on your journey toward recovery. Be determined and persistent. Stay the course.

Keep fighting for recovery,

The ARC Team
Carol, Kim, David, and Christine

Mail Donations to:
Aphasia Recovery Connection
c/o Huggins
424 2nd Street
Marietta, Ohio
45750

Introduction to ARC

Aphasia Recovery Connection

Aphasia Recovery Connection (ARC) is an award-winning non-profit organization that works to help end the isolation for people recovering from aphasia. This book is designed to help families navigate the road to recovery as they gain an understanding of aphasia, review various rehab options, and discover ways to maximize their recovery potential.

ARC : *For* Families Dealing with Aphasia

By Families Dealing with Aphasia

ARC was started in 2012 by young stroke survivors Christine Huggins and David Dow with the help of David's mom, Carol, who serves as its Director. It started as a simple Facebook group but quickly grew into the fastest growing aphasia support group online, serving thousands. Months later, their website, aphasiarecoveryconnection.org, went up and the buzz in the aphasia world began.

Soon the dynamic duo, along with their moms, were leading aphasia conferences, retreats, cruises, video calls, and adding support groups specific to caregivers, pediatric aphasia families, and more. In

2013, they received a *RAISE Award* from the National Stroke Association for making an impact on the lives of stroke survivors.

ARC presented at the American Speech-Language-Hearing Association (ASHA) Conferences in 2013 and 2014. ARC leaders are in-demand speakers. They have given presentations at aphasia centers, support groups, and recently at the Rehabilitation Institute of Chicago. Christine and David were the keynote speakers for the Ohio Governor's Council Youth Leadership Forum.

ARC's success is often summed up by its members who say, "ARC gets it." ARC "gets it" because they live it. The team believes there are three main experts on aphasia: the therapists and medical personnel, the person with aphasia, and the families. ARC successfully brings the synergy and cooperation of the groups together, which serves to help families who are often struggling with the same issues we have.

The ARC Leadership Team

Founders David and Christine are the heart and soul of ARC. They have walked the road to recovery with bumps, successes, failures, tears, grief, laughter and hope along the way. They have walked in your shoes. The goal of this book is to offer you a companion on your own road to recovery.

Christine Huggins was working as an attorney when a stroke interrupted her life in 2011, at age twenty six, due to to an undetected hole in her heart. She has actively worked on her recovery for years and has developed many ARC programs including the ARC website, video chats, and their popular Pinterest site. She is also serving on the Ohio Governor's Council for People with Disabilities.

David Dow suffered a massive stroke at age ten in 1995. He was hospitalized for three months due to a rare vascular defect called moyamoya. Since then, David has had over 15 years of speech therapy, with nearly 50 speech therapists. He's been featured in People Magazine, on Good Morning America, and has written a book, ***"Brain Attack: My Journey of Recovery from Stroke and Aphasia."*** It is an aphasia-friendly easy read available on Amazon.

Their moms, Carol and Kim, have nearly 25 years of combined aphasia recovery experiences as caregivers. They are active advocates for those dealing with this devastating disability.

Kim Huggins brings her experience as a primary grade school teacher, which has been invaluable to Christine's recovery as well as to ARC members online who benefit from her weekly "Tips from Mrs. Hugg." She's also developed several recovery teaching techniques that have helped Christine and ARC members such as the "Hugg Method" and her "Stretch a Sentence" which she teaches at ARC events. Kim is currently working on developing educational modules for ARC's Aphasia U, launching in 2015. Christine's dad, an attorney, helped ARC with their plans as they worked to become a nationally recognized non-profit organization.

Carol Dow-Richards (co-author of this book) is ARC's Director and has been an advocate for people with aphasia for over twenty years as a writer and public speaker. She facilitates four support groups in Las Vegas and connects with families dealing with aphasia on a daily basis. Carol works passionately to engage people with aphasia in their recoveries, working to instill motivation and hope.

Carol's older son, Dr. Mike Dow, is a psychotherapist with expertise in brain health, and a regular guest on TV shows such as *Dr. Oz* and *The Doctors*. His insight has helped his family understand the value of looking at the whole person in body, mind, and spirit, as they've each walked their own recovery journey. Mike serves on the advisory board for Aphasia U Boot Camp.

ARC Activities

The ARC Facebook sites offer not only written postings but also features many videos from the ARC team as well as from some of the top aphasia experts in the country. A sampling of recent topics include: recovery outcomes for people with aphasia, how to type on the phone without spelling, information about aphasia for family members, and information about new apps for aphasia.

Video posts are helpful for those who have difficulty reading due to their aphasia. Videos provide both visual and auditory information making the material more accessible for those with aphasia. Videos also allow for pausing and playback to enhance comprehension.

The ARC Facebook Page

The public site is for those interested in aphasia. It offers many videos as well as educational posters for people with aphasia to share on their own time lines.   **facebook.com/aphasiaARC**

The ARC Facebook Group

The private site is for people with aphasia, their loved ones, and related professionals. It is not open to the general public and only members can see posts. You can request membership at:

facebook.com/groups/Aphasia.Recovery.Connection

ARC Aphasia Cruises

ARC Aphasia Cruises are offered every year for people with aphasia and their families. Educational sessions are offered onboard daily by Speech Therapists and the ARC leadership team. The group dines together every evening. ARC cruises are a popular choice for people who want to meet others with aphasia while vacationing. David shares, "There are no taxis, unpacking at every location, and it is so much easier with my physical disabilities to be on a ship." For the latest cruise offerings, email David at ARCaphasia@gmail.com

ARC Retreats

ARC Retreats offer families dealing with aphasia a place to meet and share their experiences with other families. For more information on ARC Retreats, visit our website or email Kim at ARCaphasia@gmail.com

ARC Aphasia U Boot Camp

ARC Aphasia U Boot Camp is launching in 2015. These intensive aphasia educational and social immersion programs will offer attendees a safe place to practice new skills, meet others, share stories, explore options and set goals for their continued journey on their road to recovery. Topics will include technology, motivation, coping, insurance issues, making friends, and communication strategies. Located in Las Vegas, the program will also offer attendees a chance for fun and social engagement as the group has excursions together.

Boot Camp will provide video teaching modules by some of the leading experts in recovery today from speech therapists, aphasia companies, psychotherapists, social workers, medical doctors, people living with aphasia and more. (This is not a medical model and will not be covered by insurance.) ARC aims to make Boot Camp a way to optimize recovery using the Life Participation Approach to Aphasia. Space is limited. For more information email Carol at: ARCaphasia@gmail.com

ARC - Where Making a Difference Matters

ARC gets messages of appreciation daily from family members. Aphasia is a lonely place, but it doesn't have to be. As one ARC member shared, there is value in connecting people with aphasia: "My loved one was struggling to cope and was feeling hopeless. Then she attended an ARC event and met others with aphasia. She had given up.

Now she is back at therapy and she is trying again. Thank you for instilling hope. We thought she'd lost that."

About the Authors

Carol Dow-Richards is the Director of the Aphasia Recovery Connection. She holds a B.S. in Psychology and has worked as a public school teacher with a focus on language-based learning disabilities.

Amanda Anderson is a Speech and Language Pathologist who specializes in publications for people with aphasia. She is the author of several aphasia workbooks (see page 150) that David and Christine use. While completing her Masters at the University of Hawaii, she was one of David's student clinicians when he was 8 years post stroke.

Amanda's workbooks (Speech Therapy Aphasia Rehabilitation *STAR* Workbooks) caught the attention of the Aphasia Recovery Connection's leadership team. They were impressed with how easy they are to use, helping people with aphasia optimize recovery in therapy and on their own at home. With over 18 years of speech therapy under his belt, you can imagine how many aphasia workbooks and therapy tools David has used. David and Carol love Amanda's books and use them in many of their communication groups and ARC activities. People with aphasia share how helpful her workbooks are especially with continuing progress once speech therapy insurance benefits have run out. They include many of the helpful aphasia therapy techniques discussed in this book.

The Book

David and Amanda reconnected after ten years. They discovered they were both authors with a passion for making a difference for those struggling to cope with aphasia. It was David's suggestion that Amanda work with ARC on a book. She quickly agreed not only to help ARC with their first book, but also to donate all proceeds to Aphasia Recovery Connection.

This book started with David's suggestion that people with aphasia needed a concierge. David explained that a concierge in a hotel helps people figure out what to do, where to go, and how to best budget their time and money while in a new city. He thinks people with aphasia need that same type of help. They need to know what the options are and how to best budget their time and resources. There are so many options that it becomes overwhelming for people as they ponder a multitude of choices.

They wonder what insurance covers and what it doesn't. They may want to meet others with aphasia online or in person. Should they attend an ARC Aphasia Retreat? Do they want to experience ARC's Aphasia U Boot Camp in Las Vegas?

Should they choose teletherapy online via a webcam or face-to-face therapy? Perhaps they are looking for activities, apps, or workbooks to supplement their therapy hours to enhance recovery.

Some people can afford all of the options, but many are left to wonder what they should devote their resources to. They don't want to make a misstep on the journey but find themselves confused as to where they should prioritize their spending. If they have little to no funds at all, they need to know how to maximize their insurance or perhaps find options with free therapy clinics or clinical trials.

Sometimes they just need a good cry and to know they aren't alone. Knowing there are others out there you can reach out to is invaluable. ARC's primary mission is to end the isolation of aphasia.

"We need to help people like the hotel concierge,
who helps people learn their options, costs,
and what the best options are
based on their own needs and budget.
People with aphasia need a road map."
-David Dow

So with that, we got to work. This book provides information about aphasia and the different options available to supplement your speech and language rehabilitation. We are not endorsing any particular method or idea. We're just letting you know your choices and helping you learn more so you can make smart decisions along your own road to recovery.

Disclaimer

The information and advice provided here is not meant as medical advice in any way. The recommendations provided are for informational purposes only. We encourage readers to consult a medical professional before beginning any course of action based on the topics covered within this book.

Reading this book

We understand that many people with aphasia will be unable to read this book. However, we are hoping that family members can read some portions of it to the person with aphasia. Speech-Language Pathologists might also utilize it for reading practice with their patients.

AN INVISIBLE DISABILITY

APHASIA

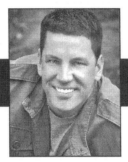

speaking

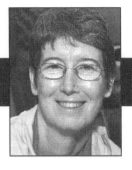

reading

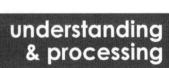

writing

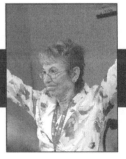

understanding & processing

ARC members with aphasia

Chapter 1

Aphasia: The Basics

Aphasia is a neurological disorder resulting from damage to the language centers of the brain. Aphasia is an invisible yet devastating disability. People with aphasia may have difficulty with speaking (expressive language), understanding (receptive language), or both. Writing, reading, and math may also be challenging for people with aphasia. Aphasia is a language disorder and can mask a person's intelligence.[i]

Often, people with aphasia are mistaken for being intellectually disabled. However, they are indeed thinking and are still smart. You know you are still smart but sometimes others may not understand that because you are having difficulty communicating. Aphasia can be so frustrating and initially, you may be overwhelmed by the changes. Co-author, Carol Dow-Richards says, " I often explain it to loved ones or audiences like this: If I were to place someone on an island where they did not speak, read, write, or understand the language, would their own intellect be affected? That often gives families a better understanding of aphasia.

Anything that causes damage to the language centers of the brain can cause aphasia. The most common cause of aphasia is a stroke. Aphasia can also result from other conditions that can cause a brain injury such as infection, head injury, aneurism, dementia, or brain tumors.[ii]

Strokes

Strokes are the leading cause of aphasia. There are various types of strokes. It is important to know why you had a stroke to better understand both treatment options as well as to learn ways to reduce your risks of future strokes.

Ischemic strokes are caused by blood clots that obstruct blood flow to the brain and make up 87% of all stroke cases.[iii] When brain cells stop receiving blood rich in oxygen, even for a few minutes, the cells will die.

Ischemic strokes can be either thrombotic or embolic. Thrombotic strokes result from a buildup of fatty tissue in arteries in the brain, sometimes where the artery has already begun to narrow. This blockage can stop adequate blood supply to language centers of the brain.

Embolic strokes are caused by clots in arteries that formed somewhere else in the body, such as the heart. Part of the clot can break off and travel to the brain, causing a blockage and an ischemic stroke.[iv]

Hemorrhagic strokes cause the remaining 13% of strokes.[v] This occurs when an artery inside the brain ruptures. The bleeding causes increased swelling and pressure in the brain resulting in damaged brain cells.[vi] Bleeding can be caused by aneurysm and arteriovenous malformation (AVM). An arteriovenous malformation is "a cluster of abnormally formed blood vessels" which are vulnerable to breaking and bleeding.[vii] An aneurysm is a balloon-like pouch on an artery that weakens and can eventually burst.

Carotid and vertebral artery dissections are causes of stroke that are difficult to prevent. Trauma or underlying congenital weakness causes the layers of the carotid or vertebral artery to tear and bleed. The interior lining of the artery then bulges out which can cause blockage of blood flow to the brain.

Carotid and vertebral artery dissections are a leading cause of strokes in younger patients. Chiropractic neck adjustments, looking up for an extended period of time, roller coaster rides, car accidents, violent coughing spells, vomiting and even blowing up a balloon can cause carotid artery dissections.

Aphasia

Every year over 200,000 people in the United States are diagnosed with aphasia.[viii] Aphasia is more prevalent than Parkinson's Disease, Muscular Dystrophy, and Cerebral Palsy, yet most people have never heard of it.[ix] Between 25% and 40% of stroke survivors have some form of aphasia.[x]

Carol Dow-Richards explains, "When David had his stroke, we found ourselves very frustrated and afraid, terrified really. Initially the doctors didn't explain aphasia to us as they were concentrating on saving his life and limiting the damage from the stroke. As he lay in bed unable to speak, read, write, or even understand, I wondered, *Is there any hope? Is aphasia permanent? How do people deal with this?*"

Some people leave the hospital without an understanding of aphasia. Some aren't even sure what their language impairment is called, making it difficult to search for information and get help.

Your Recovery Team

There is an entire professional field dedicated to helping you recover. You may have several doctors and specialists working with you.

Physical Therapists (PTs) help with gross motor (large motor) rehabilitation. They may help with fitting you with a wheelchair, walking, and keeping you safe while you adapt to any paralysis you may have.

Occupational Therapists (OTs) help with fine motor (small motor) rehabilitation. The OT may help you adapt to being one handed if you have one-sided weakness which is called hemiparesis. They also work to help restore function to the use of your weakened hand and arm. OTs also work with activities of daily living such as bathing and dressing.

Speech-Language Pathologists (SLPs) help you recover your expressive language (talking), receptive language (understanding), reading, and writing function. They can also treat any swallowing disorders (dysphagia) that you may have. Speech-Language Pathologists are sometimes referred to as speech therapists.

You and your loved ones are also big players on the team. Just like with a sports team where players work cooperatively, rest and motivation are big factors in a team's success. Staying engaged in your rehabilitation is a way to maximize your ability to make the best recovery possible.

A Speech-Language Pathologist will evaluate you to determine your type of aphasia. No two cases of aphasia are exactly alike. The part of your brain that was damaged is called a lesion. The size and location of your brain lesion will determine what type of language deficits you have. You might want to ask your doctor to show you your brain scans so you can see the area and have a better understanding of what happened.

You should not compare yourself to others you meet with aphasia because lesions vary greatly as do types of aphasia. Some people may be able to read, but not talk. Most people with aphasia have some difficulty with word finding but some can write while others can't. For some, talking is easier but they may have difficulty understanding. Others will have all of the problems associated with aphasia. The good news is most people with aphasia will continue to recover and your aphasia will never be as bad as it was in the beginning.

Receptive Aphasia

Aphasia can impair receptive language. This makes understanding others challenging. Wernicke's aphasia, fluent aphasia or receptive aphasia all refer to types of aphasia with comprehension deficits. Somebody with receptive aphasia may have difficulty understanding what others are saying or may need extra time to process spoken words in order to increase comprehension. Background noise, visual distractions, and multiple speakers can make comprehension for somebody with aphasia even more challenging.

In some cases, a person with aphasia may have no trouble getting words out, but the words they use are incorrect and they often use made-up words. A person with this type of aphasia usually has difficulty recognizing that what they are saying is incorrect.

Stroke survivor, Lisa Wagner, shared her experience when she first realized that she had aphasia, *"I think I talk right, but most people had no clue what I was saying. Why would someone not tell me this? They were all so nice, nodding heads and smiling, so I thought I am fine...."* She wasn't fine. Her speech had become a combination of made up words and she wasn't able to recognize her errors because of both expressive and receptive aphasia. [xi]

Expressive Aphasia

Expressive aphasia can range from severe, where the person is only able to say only a few words, to mild aphasia with occasional word finding difficulties (anomia). Anomia is the sensation of having the word on the tip of your tongue but not quite being able to say the word.

Expressive aphasia often limits a person's ability to participate in conversations and express basic wants and needs. Aphasia can be extremely isolating. The following are all different names for types of expressive aphasia: Non-fluent Aphasia, Broca's Aphasia, Transcortical Motor Aphasia, Conduction Aphasia, and Anomic Aphasia.[xii] They are all caused by damage to Broca's area of the brain.

Global Aphasia

Global aphasia is the most severe type of aphasia because it combines both difficulty talking and understanding. Global aphasia is typical of somebody who has endured a severe stroke or brain injury that has damaged multiple areas of the brain.

David was diagnosed with global aphasia. He had difficulty with math, talking, understanding, reading, writing and even gesturing. With the help of SLPs and a lot of hard work, today he talks, understands, reads, and writes and is a professional public speaker! People with aphasia can and do improve. It takes work. There is no magic pill.

Christine also had global aphasia. She recalls lying in the hospital bed and wanting someone to bring her eyeglasses to the hospital. No one did. They didn't realize they were missing (she usually wore contacts) and Christine was unable to verbalize or even gesture that she wanted them. Without her glasses, she was unable to see well, so she also had difficulty looking for facial expressions or cues to help her understand what people were trying to tell her.

Characteristics of Aphasia

In the beginning, it is important to know what you are able to do and what types of communication are difficult. Some people with aphasia can write what they want to say while others have just as much difficulty with writing as they do with speaking. If you are able to write, do it! Using communication in any form will be beneficial for your recovery.

Some people with aphasia can repeat words after they hear them, while others have difficulty with repetition.[xiii] If you are able to repeat after hearing a word or sentence, this is an excellent way to practice improving your expressive language function.

Some of the frustrating symptoms of aphasia include:

Anomia: Difficulty with word finding.

Semantic Paraphasia: Substituting an incorrect word for another with or without recognizing the mistake.

Phonemic Paraphasia: Substituting, adding, or rearranging the speech sounds in a word.

Jargon: Fluent utterances that make little or no sense, often seen in receptive aphasia.[xiv]

Perseveration: Getting stuck on a previous word and saying it over and over despite a new topic or question.

Circumlocutions: Talking around a word. Describing and using other words to explain what you are trying to say. This is actually a very positive technique and is encouraged as a compensatory strategy.

Acalculia: Loss of ability to complete mathematical calculations.

Agrammatism: Utterances that are missing the appropriate parts of speech.

Neologistic paraphasia: spoken words that are made up. For example: wonkerblat for shirt.

Apraxia and Dysarthria

People with aphasia may also have other motor speech disorders, such as apraxia or dysarthria.

Apraxia is a disorder that impacts the brain's ability to control and coordinate muscles required for speech. Apraxia impacts motor planning function and can make it difficult to say the correct sounds in each word.

Dysarthria is a deficit that causes slurred speech secondary to oral and lingual (tongue) muscle weakness. Somebody with aphasia may present with difficulties in multiple areas or just one, depending on the size and location of the lesion caused by their brain injury.

Carol Dow-Richards recalls, David's first sentence was months after his stroke. "He suffered from both of dysarthria and apraxia as well. We had gone thru a drive-thru window and I handed him his food. *Ank ou om,* he said. I remember being thrilled to hear a three-word sentence, *Thank you mom*. Progress was slow, but it was indeed progress."

Recovery Times

Just as the severity and type of aphasia vary from person to person, so will recovery. Many factors determine how well someone with aphasia will be able to recover including the size and location of the brain lesion, family support, age, motivation, amount of social interaction, prior activity level, and access to therapy.

Spontaneous recovery occurs within the first few hours and days after a stroke or brain injury. This is a result of the reduction of swelling in the brain, neuroplasticity, and overall restoration of tissue function in the brain.[xv] As your body recovers in the first few days, you may see a dramatic increase in speech and language function. Also, changes in metabolism and reduction of abnormalities of blood flow caused by the stroke or brain injury help promote spontaneous recovery.[xvi]

The next few weeks are considered the subacute phase where the brain begins to form new neural connections and begins neural reorganization to help speech and language recovery.[xvii]

The chronic phase of recovery can last anywhere from a few months to years and even decades.[xviii] The National Stroke Association states, "A full recovery from aphasia is possible, but if symptoms persist long enough, usually more than six months, then a complete recovery becomes unlikely."[xix] Improvement varies from person to person but recovery has been noted to occur long after the initial stroke or brain injury. The National Aphasia Association states that recovery from aphasia can occur over a period of years or even decades.[xx] David's most dramatic gains came nearly six years after his stroke.

Many members of Aphasia Recovery Connection have shared that they have experienced continued gains many years after their diagnosis of aphasia. Connie Snell remarks on her husband's continued progress with speech therapy and says, "It will be two years since my husband's stroke. He has been in speech therapy the entire time and we are still seeing notable improvement."

Christine has improved significantly long after her insurance-covered therapy ended. She works daily to improve her skills and fights for recovery every single day, sometimes working for several hours on skills that challenge her brain. She says, "It is like a workout everyday. It is tiring, but I must do it."

Benefits of Speech Therapy

The American Speech-Language-Hearing Association (ASHA) states that both clinical and research findings point to the benefits of speech therapy to improve communication function for individuals with aphasia. A research study by Wertz R. T. et al. shows that people with aphasia who receive "8-10 hours of treatment each week for 12 weeks make significantly greater improvement than individuals with aphasia who are not treated." [xxi]

The American Speech-Language-Hearing Association collects outcome measures on results from speech therapy with people with aphasia. Their data shows that approximately 80% of stroke patients with receptive and expressive language disorders make significant improvement with speech therapy.[xxii]

Hope

Although aphasia is a very complex and difficult language disability, there is hope. Over the last decade, there has been a multitude of research on the brain's ability to repair itself. Everyday on ARC's Facebook site, people at various stages on the road to recovery share stories of improvement. While it is a challenging path, it is one full of gains and gradual success.

We invite you to join us on the Aphasia Recovery Connection Facebook group site. You will meet others, be able to learn and share your experiences, ask questions, and most of all you'll find a group who is positive, hopeful and caring. You can find instructions on how to join our Facebook group in Appendix C on page 144 of this book.

Bloom Where You Are Planted – David Dow

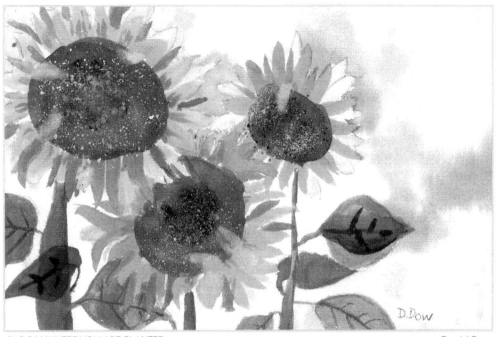

BLOOM WHERE YOU ARE PLANTED   David Dow

Think Positive. I am unable to use my right hand at all. I painted this with my left hand. I gave it a title. *Bloom Where You Are Planted.* None of us wanted a stroke or aphasia but we have it, so we have to do our best.

        -David Dow

Chapter 2

Aphasia: In the Hospital

A person who has had a stroke typically spends an average of six days in the hospital.[xxiii] This will vary depending on the severity of the stroke or brain injury and what type of medical care is needed. Patients who are medically stable may start to receive rehabilitation therapy as soon as two days after their stroke.[xxiv]

David required brain surgery that resulted in nearly three months of hospitalization. Christine also needed surgery but it is important that you don't compare yourself to other people. Your case is uniquely yours.

The initial shock of realizing you are unable to communicate can be terrifying. Your body is still in shock from the injury to your brain. You might not be able to figure out how to communicate with the nursing staff or family. Honestly, they may not be sure how to best communicate with you, either. Not all nursing staff have had training to understand aphasia.

Christine Huggins, Co-Founder of ARC, had difficulty communicating after her stroke. She recalls, "I was thirsty. SO thirsty and I did not have a communication board and I could not spell." At the time, Christine remembers wanting a paper and pen. She was sure she could draw a picture of a cup that would show the staff what she needed but since she could not tell them with words, she waited a long time for a drink of water.

Christine is very smart but those first few days with aphasia were very disorienting. She realized later that maybe she could have gestured for a glass of water. She remembers that staff seemed to rush in and out. She needed more time and patience from them so she could explain what she needed. It is very common for patients to find these first few days a blur of activity and confusion and like many people with aphasia, she did not realize that her sentences were not making sense to anyone.

Carol Dow-Richards recalls being in the ICU with David: "I was sure he understood. I really believed we'd be home soon and he would be fine. I think that was my way of coping as it was too much to deal with. Often denial becomes a way to cope but eventually we had to accept that his aphasia was not going away anytime soon. We had a very long road ahead of us."

People with aphasia need patience. They need staff with an understanding of aphasia and how to communicate with them. Patients need tools to help them communicate but from what we hear from most ARC members, tools such as communication boards or even smartphone apps are rarely used and staff have limited time.

On the following page is a very basic communication board to help you during your hospital and rehab stay. You can use the picture communication board from the book or have somebody make a copy so you can point to the pictures. See if you can get a clipboard so you can keep the communication board with you. There are also communication board apps for your smartphone, some are even free. To find them, use the search terms "communication board aphasia." There are versions for both smartphones and tablets.

Basic Communication Board

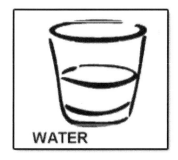

WATER

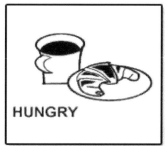

HUNGRY

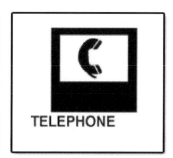

TELEPHONE

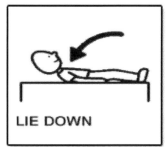

LIE DOWN

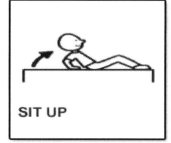

SIT UP

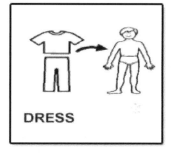

DRESS

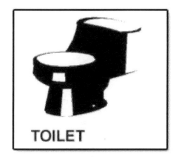

TOILET

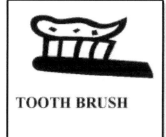

TOOTH BRUSH

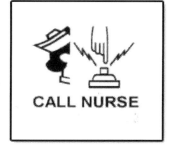

CALL NURSE

SHOWER

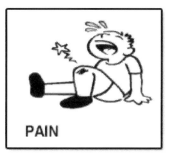

PAIN

YES

NO

33

ARC member Lisa describes her experience in the hospital:

"Tankfew." I said. My nurse responded, "What?" *Sigh. "Blysiy tankfew."* My hand reach my chest and pat my heart. My husband added, *"She's saying thank you."* *"Oh you're welcome, hon,"* my nurse replied on her way out the door. I think, *"My name is not hon. My name Lisa. Can't she read the stupid sign on the door? Why can't I talk? What happen to me? Why am I lying in bed and not home? John is here. What the hell is going on?"*

Later my nurse returned, "Time to draw more blood, hon. How are WE today? I think, *"How are we? Really?? Let's see, I not able to talk, the doctor keep saying I have a stroke and it might take time to talk again, IF at all. So WE are scared to tears, can't do anything and stuck in bed with YELLOW socks on and not allowed up. That how WE are today. But in fact I just try to be calm and let her draw my blood and leave.* As the nurse leave I say to her, *"Ru nraw dreff. Nraw maa."* "What?" *Sigh.* I meant to say, *"I'm not deaf do not yell at me and leave me alone."* I remember John said to her, "She said thank you."

Another ARC member shared that he pressed the nurse's button and heard the response, "Can I help you?" *Silence-he could not talk. He pressed it again. Silence. He tried again and again.* Finally a nurse came to his room and he was met with tremendous anger, "Do NOT press the button again and again. TALK into the microphone." She demonstrated it and stormed out of his room. *He could NOT talk. He did have needs. Important needs. Human needs. He wet himself. Left to feel humiliated and disgraced, misunderstood and frustrated, he cried.*

ARC member Charade describes how she discovered she was having trouble with her receptive and expressive language. She explains, *"Well, I thought that I spoke fine after my stroke. I thought that my family, my doctors, nurses, physical therapist, occupational therapist and my best friends were talking different tongue, like a Punk TV show. I didn't want a speech therapist. I studied AP English and AP history. My right side was disabled not my speech.*

After 2 weeks, when my father visited me, I decided to tell

everyone there hey speak English please I was bothered about the

different language. I spoke English and Spanish fluently, I read

Spanish and English, and write well. So I tell my father, about

that, and he didn't understand. He looked sad, and he wrote you

have aphasia. I was puzzled, he explained speech disorder, and he

told my speech is mumbles and everyone couldn't understand my

speech. I was ashamed. I was very confused, and I cried and I will

not speak anymore. However I read, my dream world.

There is additional education that needs to take place to
inform hospital staff about aphasia. Sometimes patients may not
recall being told they have aphasia. Some are not told or if they are
it may be so brief that they are unsure how to spell aphasia to
research at home.

ARC member Thomas shared his story with ARC: *I never*

knew about aphasia until about a year ago when I saw a video

with a young lady that talks like me. I didn't know there is a word

for that! It had been 14 years and there is a word for that!?! I

really gave my doctor heck when I saw her the next time. She

apologized and said that it is only a part of the problems that I have from my head injury and she didn't know it would mean that much to me. Then, she started telling me about different forms of aphasia and I got confused again!

Even medical staff have difficulty understanding the needs of somebody with aphasia. Carol Dow-Richards recalls visiting an ARC member when suddenly he was unable to use his right leg and the left side of his face drooped. They rushed to the ER knowing these were classic stroke symptoms.

In the ER, the doctor started rattling off information very quickly so Carol said, "He has aphasia." The doctor continued on at the same speed, seemingly ignoring me or perhaps he not knowing how to adapt his communication style for a patient with aphasia. Next, a technician came in and the scene was repeated and then again with a nurse.

Unfortunately lack of understanding of aphasia seems to be the norm according to experiences shared by ARC members. Carol has been in the ER seven different times with different people with aphasia and advocating for them has been necessary every single time.

She went to the nurses' station and asked for a piece of paper, a clipboard, and pen and wrote this down for her friend:

– **I have aphasia.**

– **I worked as an engineer.**

– **Aphasia does not affect my intellect.**

– **Please reduce your rate of speech.**

– **Emphasize key words.**

– **I can read. Write down key words.**

– **I communicate with a whiteboard app on my iPad.**

Every time Carol visited him over the next week, he proudly showed her the clipboard he kept in bed with him and he would give her a 'high five.' After he was discharged from the hospital he and his wife sent Carol a photo of him holding up the clipboard, pointing to it, with a thumbs up. He was so thankful to have this simple reference to show the staff. It empowered him to self advocate and enhanced communication with staff and visitors.

You might adapt this example for your own use during your hospital stay. If you are not in the hospital as you read this, you can still make a communication list and keep it handy. This way, if you ever return to the ER or when you visit a doctor's office, you are able to advocate for your own needs by sharing information.

It is remarkable what a few pieces of information about aphasia can do to improve communication. In Appendix A on page 142, you'll find a template to complete with your own information. You may want to ask your Speech-Language Pathologist to help you. You could also add other information you want people to know.

The first few days with aphasia are naturally confusing, scary, and exhausting. You may feel trapped and frustrated because of your inability to communicate. We have provided questions in bold print you can point to and use to communicate with nursing staff and caregivers. Try your best to use any modality of communication that is available to you: Nod "yes" or "no", point, make facial expressions, and use any word you can even if it isn't the exact word you want.

Ask your family member to post information about you in your room. Pictures and information about yourself can help the nursing and rehab staff know a little bit about you. Have somebody write down your interests and profession. Seeing a photo of you before your brain injury can go a long way helping nursing and rehab staff see you for who you are and not just what your medical chart says about you.

Point to the phrases below to help communicate your needs.

- **I am having trouble getting the words out.**

- **Give me a minute.**

- **I am having trouble understanding.**

- **Please use simple words.**

- **I can hear you fine. You do not need to yell.**

- **Please talk slower and explain that again.**

- **I am thirsty.**

- **I am hungry.**

- **I need to use the bathroom.**

- **I would like to take a shower.**

- **Please repeat what you just said.**

- **Call my: wife / husband/ children / mother / father / friend**

- **I understood what you said.**

- **When will I see a speech therapist?**

- **How long will I be here?**

- **How large was my stroke? Please show me my brain scan.**

- **What medication are you giving me?**

- **I'd like to talk to somebody about insurance.**

- **Why did you give me thick liquids?**

Having written communication aids can be extremely helpful. When David was hospitalized, Carol put a poster above his bed and wrote:

— David has aphasia.
— He is in the 4th grade.
— He was in the gifted program and loved to play soccer.
— He communicates his needs by head nodding – yes or no.
— He has difficulty understanding speech.
— Go slow. Keep it simple.
— His mom's name is Carol.
— David loves his dog, Schroder.
  David cannot speak at this time.

Writing

It is important to determine if you are able to write. If so, this is a fantastic mode of communication and you should use it as much as possible. Writing may actually help with your rehabilitation and will not hinder your future ability to regain verbal communication skills. If you haven't had a chance to see if you can write, now is the time! Call for your nurse or caregiver and point to the sentence below.

• ***Please bring me some paper and a pen.***

First, try writing your name. If you are unable to write your name, try writing the numbers 1 through 10. If you can write your name, practice writing your address, your phone number and other personal information. Also, try writing communication phrases such as, "Hi, how are you?" Try copying the phrase: "**I have aphasia.**"

Your Rehabilitation Team

The rehabilitation department at the hospital will evaluate you to decide what type of therapy you will need. ADLs is a term used often in rehab and it refers to any "activities of daily living" that you need assistance with in therapy.

A *Speech-Language Pathologist (*SLP) will be the professional to help you with your communication. Speech-Language Pathologists work with people with aphasia as well as apraxia, dysarthria, and dysphagia which can all result from a stroke or brain injury. A Speech -Language Pathologist has a Master's degree in communication science and is trained to evaluate and treat all communication and swallowing disorders. As you recover, you will probably work with several SLPs in different settings.

The *Physical Therapist* concentrates on gross motor (large motor) function and will help with balance, walking, and strengthening exercises. Physical therapists focus on fall prevention and help you adjust to any weakness.

The *Occupational Therapist* works with fine motor muscles (small motor) and will help with ADLs such as bathing, dressing, and safety issues. An occupational therapist will also address any weakness or contractions you have in your arms or hands.

During the first week or so, the therapists will help determine what types of assistive devices you may need. These may include a wheelchair, bedside commode, walker, cane, reacher, splint, and so on.

Physical Therapists and occupational therapists both typically have assistants. Physical therapy assistants (PTAs) and certified occupational therapy assistants (COTAs) will work with you on therapy goals. Physical Therapists and occupational therapists have at least a Master's degree and PTAs and COTAs require an Associates degree.

Typically the physical therapist and occupational therapist will do the evaluation to determine what exercises are needed to help you reach your goals and the PTAs and COTAs will help you with the exercises to reach the goals. If any changes to your treatment plan are needed, the evaluating therapist will do a re-certification to update your goals and treatment plan. Every evaluation done by a therapist requires a written doctor's order.

Swallowing

Difficulty swallowing is called dysphagia. As many as 65% of stroke survivors have dysphagia.[xxv] Strokes and brain injuries can cause damage to the nerves and muscles that control swallowing. Swallowing disorders are very serious because if you get food or liquid in your airway (trachea) and into your lungs it can cause aspiration pneumonia. Weakened swallowing function can also result in food lodging in your airway causing choking and possibly death.

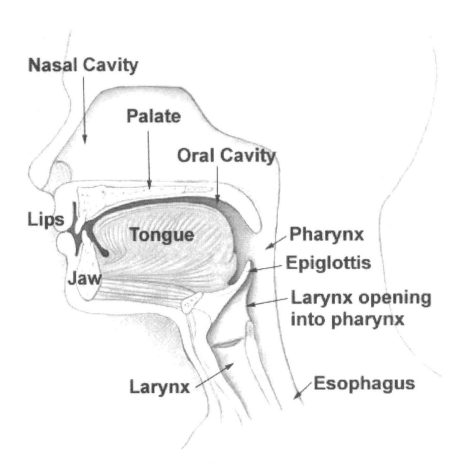

Nasal Cavity

Palate

Oral Cavity

Lips

Tongue

Pharynx

Epiglottis

Jaw

Larynx opening into pharynx

Larynx

Esophagus

xxvi

Refer to this diagram to understand the swallow process. In a normal swallow, the food or bolus travels through the oral cavity until it hits the back of the tongue and triggers the swallow reflex. The epiglottis closes to protect the larynx and the bolus travels safely into the esophagus.

Stroke survivors experience a variety of dysphagia symptoms that can result in food or liquid falling into the larynx and down into the airway and lungs, which is called aspiration. Coughing, wet vocal quality after a swallow, tearing eyes and runny noses are all signs and symptoms of aspiration. Strokes can weaken the muscles in the throat, making it difficult to clear food out of the pharynx. Damage from a brain injury can cause the epiglottis to move slower and thin liquids (regular liquids) can spill down into the trachea before the epiglottis has completely protected the airway.

Some stroke and brain injury survivors are given the status NPO which means "nothing by mouth" and may need a feeding tube to safely obtain nutrition and hydration. Others will need thickened liquids in order to allow enough time to swallow safely and prevent liquids from entering your airway. Keep in mind, just because you are having trouble swallowing right after your stroke and doctors recommend a feeding tube doesn't mean it will be permanent.

Your first encounter with a Speech-Language Pathologist may be during a bedside swallow evaluation to determine what you can safely eat and drink. They may request a doctor's order for a Modified Barium Swallow (MBS) which is a video X-ray of your swallow. A MBS will show whether or not you are aspirating (food or liquids going down the wrong way).

Your SLP will show you what types of exercises you need to do to strengthen your swallowing muscles and increase your safety and swallow function. Dysphagia typically takes priority over aphasia therapy and your SLP will focus on making sure you can eat and drink without the risk of choking or aspirating. It is a good idea to think of your SLP as a coach guiding you through the recovery process. They have the tools to teach you how to improve and ideally they can show you what you need to do on your own to optimize your recovery. Here are some questions you can ask your SLP:

— *What exercises can I do on my own to improve swallowing?*

— *What can I start to do on my own to improve communication?*

— *Can you show my family how to work with me on my goals?*

Visitors

You may be eager to see family and friends and also have some concerns about how they will react to your aphasia. Immediately after a stroke or brain injury you will be understandably tired and fatigue easily. Your body needs sleep to help repair and recover. Aphasia symptoms can worsen when you are tired or stressed.

When you have visitors you might want to consider the following tips to improve communication:

- Reduce background noise.
- Keep the visits short.
- Turn off the TV.
- Have only one visitor at at time to eliminate side conversations.
- Avoid visits before or right after therapy.
- Evenings and weekends are ideal times for visitors.
- Ask visitors to bring photos, magazines, music or games so you can enjoy visiting with less focus on talking.

There is no right or wrong way to handle visitors. Do what will be best for you and your family. What will help optimize progress? What would you like to do and who would you like to see and when? Consider your emotional needs as well.

Family members also can play a role in helping you recover. Kim Huggins, Christine's mom, shares that she found that smiling and getting Christine's attention before she began to speak was helpful to improve comprehension. She found that speaking slower and pausing between sentences, emphasizing and writing key words, and drawing were helpful for communication. She added, "Of course family members cannot do this all day long, but I could do this during the day to help improve communication with Christine."

Aphasia is much more than language loss. For most people there is a tremendous emotional struggle as they try to cope as a family with the life obstacles that come along with aphasia.

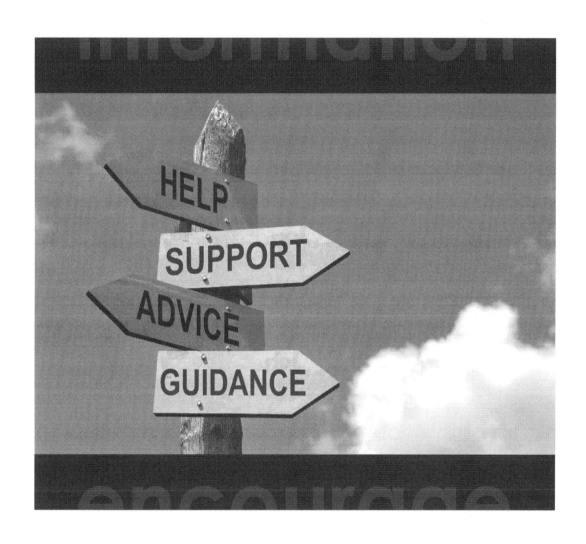

Chapter 3

Rehabilitation Options

Leaving the Hospital

Your journey of recovery is just beginning when you leave the hospital. The severity of your lesion and your physical limitations will determine where you go when you leave. While many patients look forward to discharge, it is important to remember that the road to recovery can be a long one. Some people with aphasia are able to go home, others go to rehab hospitals, assisted living facilities or skilled nursing facilities.

The severity of your disabilities and your physical limitations will be determining factors your rehab team considers when making their rehabilitation setting recommendations. Wherever you go, the therapy and hard work will continue.

Many people will find that their insurance dictates the next steps of where you go and the therapy you will receive. Your rehab team and the hospital social worker will help guide you as you consider your discharge options.

Sometimes a call to your insurance company is helpful at this stage to understand the limitations of your policy. Can you travel? How many days of therapy will be covered?

In David's case, the hospital staff suggested a rehab hospital that was one of the best in the country. However, his family chose to go to a rehab hospital that was closer to their home.

Carol Dow-Richards explains, "Cost and family considerations weighed into our decision. Had we opted for the "best" that would have meant 2-3 months of added hotel, transportation, food costs as well as being away from home, my 15-year-old son, and my business. It just was not feasible and we had to face that reality."

Be honest with the hospital staff as you look at options. Do you have family dynamics or budget concerns that affect the decision? These variables are important as well. We will look at some of the various options you may be considering once you are discharged from acute care.

Rehabilitation Hospital

Rehab hospitals are devoted to patients who have stabilized their medical condition and are approved for continued care and services within an inpatient medical setting. Often they are separate facilities but occasionally they are units within a larger hospital.

While you may opt for the recommendation the staff makes, remember that you have a choice where you go for rehabilitation. You and your family are your own advocates. There are rehabilitation hospitals with special units devoted solely to stroke and brain injury rehabilitation. Even if you need to travel, it could be worth the inconvenience of a day or more of travel to reach the best rehabilitation team for your needs.

U.S News and World Report ranks the best rehabilitation hospitals in the country. In 2014, the top five were:

1. Rehabilitation Institute of Chicago

2. Kessler Institute for Rehabilitation in West Orange, NJ

3. TIRR Memorial Hermann in Houston, TX

4. University of Washington Medical Center in Seattle, WA

5. Mayo Clinic in Rochester, MN[xxvii]

The Rehabilitation Institute of Chicago has been ranked the top rehabilitation hospital in the U.S since 1999. They accept patients from all over the world and have a department to help set up referrals and assist with travel plans. The first three months after your hospitalization is when you have the most insurance coverage. If your insurance covers an out of state rehabilitation hospital, take advantage of your benefits and consider this option. The phone number for the Rehabilitation Institute of Chicago (RIC) is: 1-800-354-7342.

Ask your doctor and social worker to help refer you to a rehabilitation hospital. The social worker will help you determine what your insurance will cover. The *U.S. News and World Report* website has additional rankings of rehabilitation hospitals. There may be one close to you on the list.

health.usnews.com/best-hospitals/rankings/rehabilitation

Recently, David was the keynote speaker at the Rehabilitation Institute of Chicago's Annual Aphasia Day. RIC has an intensive aphasia program. There are several other intensive aphasia programs in the United States and Canada.

Skilled Nursing

A skilled nursing facility (SNF) cares for patients who need long-term nursing care or rehabilitation therapy services. Sometimes it is called a long-term care facility, nursing home, or rehab center.

If you have multiple medical needs or require physical,

occupational, and speech therapy you may decide to stay at a skilled nursing facility. You may have a choice in where you go for therapy. If you are considering a SNF, you can have a friend or loved one visit several to help you decide.

If you have the luxury of having somebody tour skilled nursing facilities for you, there are some important things they should look for and questions they should ask on your behalf. How many hours a week can you expect to get therapy? How many years of experience does the Speech-Language Pathologist have? The abbreviation CFY stands for clinical fellowship year and means the speech therapist is in their first year out of graduate school. Sometimes this can be a positive thing because new graduates can be full of energy and motivated to give you the best therapy they can. Although, CFYs may lack the experience that may be necessary for your ideal rehabilitation.

Ask if the SNF rehab department uses graduate student clinicians. This will mean a student could be the one treating you. Also, find out if the speech therapist gives homework assignments. Express interest in wanting to continue therapy when you have family and friends visit. Ask what type of guidance they give their patients once they leave the skilled nursing setting. Do they provide a care plan for you once you return home? Some skilled nursing facilities will have the physical and/or occupational therapist visit your home and do a safety evaluation before you move back home. This is a good sign that they help you with the transition back home.

When visiting a skilled nursing facility (SNF), try to meet with the activities director. Some SNFs have an excellent working relationship between the therapy and activities departments. Goals for aphasia can be carried over into activities throughout the day with the activity and nursing staff. When touring a SNF look for:

- When touring a room, pull the safety call bell. See how long it takes the nursing staff to get to the room to make sure the resident is safe.
- How much supervision and help do the residents receive?
- Is the facility clean?
- Does the nursing staff seem content and happy?
- Are the residents involved in activities and up and about?
- Is it quiet or full of noise and distractions?
- Ask current residents about their experience.
- What type of therapy materials does the speech therapist have for aphasia treatment?
- If you have dysphagia. Ask if the speech therapist is certified in neuromuscular electrical stimulation therapy.

Hopefully you will have a chance to tour multiple facilities and pick the one that is the best fit for both your nursing and rehabilitation needs. Currently, if you have Medicare, Part A covers the cost of your first 100 days in a skilled nursing facility. One of the benefits of staying in a SNF is that the facility is motivated to give you the most therapy possible. The more therapy you receive, the more reimbursement the building will get for your stay. You may qualify for as many as 720 minutes of therapy (in at least two types of therapy) in 5 days. That is 12 hours of therapy in a work week or 2 hours and 24 minutes a day.

Unlike a rehabilitation hospital, not everybody who resides at a skilled nursing center is destined to return home. Many patients live there on a long term basis and have progressive conditions that will only get worse. People with advanced dementia and Alzheimer's disease may also reside at a skilled nursing facility. This is important to keep in mind when deciding where to go for rehabilitation. It could impact your emotional health to be in a skilled nursing facility because of the nature of some of the other patients' conditions.

Assisted Living

Assisted Living Facilities (ALFs) are residential buildings for people who require a variety of assistance throughout the day. ALFs provide meals, medical care, and assistance with activities of daily living. In some cases, an assisted living facility is a good match. Some have their own rehabilitation departments, eliminating the need to travel to outpatient therapy. Sometimes assisted living facilities are a transition between skilled nursing and home. If you have limited medical needs, an assisted living facility could be a good fit for you.

Assisted living would be a good setting for somebody who was thinking about moving to a place with additional support before their stroke or brain injury. If moving back home and living alone causes you and your family concern, assisted living could be the solution.

If you are considering assisted living, have someone meet with the rehab director for you if you can't do it yourself. Discuss insurance coverage. If you have Medicare and choose assisted living you will most likely use your Medicare part B benefits to cover therapy. Medicare Part B covers 80% of therapy costs at this time.

If you have Medicare it is very important to ask their rehabilitation director what their policy is for people who exceed their therapy caps. Medicare Part B allows $1,920 for occupational therapy and $1,920 for physical therapy and speech therapy combined. If you need both physical and speech therapy, the Medicare funds can run out very quickly.

Some companies discharge you from therapy as soon as you reach the cap, while others will work hard to file the paperwork to get approval for exceeding the therapy cap. Ask if they will work to extend your therapy beyond the Medicare caps.

Ask family and friends to contact your Senators and Representatives in Congress to express the need to eliminate the Part B therapy caps. There is an simple form on the American Speech-Language-Hearing Association's (ASHA) website they can fill out.

The therapy caps severely limit the rehabilitation potential for people with aphasia. Aphasia isn't something that can be fixed over a period of weeks. This is an important issue that you and your family can bring to the attention of Congress. Information on this issue can be found at this web address:

asha.org/advocacy/federal/cap.

When visiting an assisted living facility, meet with the speech therapist. Ask about average treatment frequencies and length of treatment times. See if volunteers come to the facility and are available to help with communication goals between your therapy sessions. Review the activity schedule and try to get a feel for how active and social the other residents are.

When touring the facility, note if the marketing director shows off the rehabilitation department or if they only mention it briefly. Ideally, you want a place that is proud of their therapy department and understands that their residents benefit greatly from all of the services it provides.

Home Health Therapy

Home care is care that is provided in your own home by licensed medical professionals such as nurses, speech, occupational or physical therapists. It may also include assistance provided by a professional caregiver for needs such as bathing or activities of daily living.

If you are able to go home, you may have the option of having therapists come to you. If it is difficult for you to travel to and from appointments, you may qualify for home health therapy. Home health can work with you on communication challenges that you experience.

There are some factors about home health care you may want to consider when deciding where to go for therapy. Home health speech therapists are paid by the visit and not by the total time they spend with you. They will receive the same reimbursement whether they spend 15 minutes or an hour with you. Let your home health therapist know you expect at least 45 minutes for each treatment session.

Home health therapists have to complete lengthy corporate paperwork for every visit. Some therapists will focus on completing the paperwork during your session, which may detract from the quality of therapy you receive.

Having speech therapy sessions in your home can help with real life situations and communicating with family and friends. It is also helpful to have therapy at home if you find fatigue is an issue. If you have obstacles getting to an outpatient clinic, home health can be a wonderful option.

Outpatient

Outpatient therapy is an option for people who are able to live at home but still need ongoing rehabilitation. Outpatient therapy clinics are available in a variety of settings. Check to see what therapists are approved providers through your insurance company.

Hospitals often have a separate outpatient rehabilitation clinic. Skilled nursing facilities have rehabilitation departments and sometimes are happy to see patients on an outpatient basis. Private practice speech therapy offices are also an option. Some private practices appear to only treat pediatric patients, but it could be worth your time to call and see if they also see adult patients or if they specialize in aphasia therapy.

Since your insurance may limit the number of visits you have with your speech therapist, finding an appropriate therapist for your aphasia is important. Key factors in selecting your speech therapist would include ensuring that they treat adults and have experience with aphasia therapy. To find a speech therapist who is certified by the American Speech-Language-Hearing Association, visit **asha.org** and under "Quick Links", click on "Find a Professional."

Telepractice

Telepractice refers to any type of therapy linking the clinician and patient through telecommunications technology.[xxviii] The American Speech-Language-Hearing Association has approved telepractice as an acceptable form of treatment. If you live in a rural area and have difficulty finding a Speech-Language Pathologist that suits your needs, you may be able to receive speech therapy via telepractice. This is also a great option if fatigue is an issue. If you have access to a webcam-equipped computer or tablet and are comfortable with videoconferencing applications such as Skype or ooVoo, telepractice may be an excellent option.

There are multiple aphasia treatment centers that offer aphasia treatment via telepractice. Not all insurance companies pay for telepractice so you should verify to make sure it is covered. You can ask for suggestions on telepractice therapists from ARC members who have tried this option. People often ask questions, get suggestions, and discuss topics on the ARC Facebook group site.

Insurance Concerns

Therapy benefits are allotted for each calendar year. Often your insurance benefits for speech therapy will run out after the first three months. Keep this in mind when you are working with your Speech-Language Pathologist and remember that you need goals and activities to help you through the remainder of the year.

Here are some questions you can ask:

- What can I do on my own once my therapy benefits run out?

- Could you make me a treatment plan for the rest of the year?

When a new calendar year begins, your therapy benefits reset. This is the time to begin therapy again which will require a new physician's prescription. Few places will treat once a week in order to ration therapy for the entire year. This is considered a red flag for insurance denial because it may appear to be maintenance therapy which is usually not covered. Once you begin therapy at the beginning of each year, try to leave with a plan to keep yourself going throughout the year.

Sometimes family members find that advocating and being the "squeaky wheel" with the insurance company, doctor, and therapist may result in an extension and approval for more services. However, this is not always the case because sometimes there are strict insurance limits on access to ongoing therapy.

Clinical Trials

Another way to get the most out of your therapy is to participate in clinical research trials. This is a way to obtain free therapy to improve your communication abilities. Visit: **clinicaltrials.gov** Type the word "aphasia" in the search box. You can search trials by location to see if there are any studies near you.

Motivation

We have found that motivation is key to a successful recovery. We believe it is important that there is a good rapport between the client and SLP. If you find yourself in a situation where you struggle to connect, it is your responsibility to self-advocate and seek another therapist. In fact, sometimes switching is a good idea as every therapist brings fresh ideas and approaches.

The next chapter will address how you can utilize your community to help improve your communication skills. Your Speech-Language Pathologist isn't the only person who can help you recover.

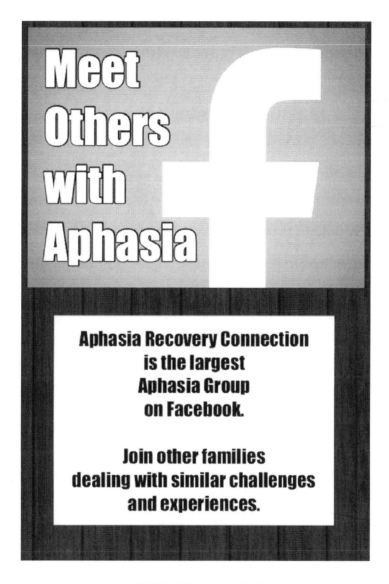

Join ARC's Facebook Group at:
www.facebook.com/groups/
Aphasia.Recovery.Connection/

Chapter 4

Circle of Support

Friends and family of someone with aphasia often want to help as much as possible, but are at a loss when it comes to knowing what to do. Since aphasia is a communication disorder, it is a challenge to let family and friends know that you want their help and to explain what they can do. Concerned family and friends sometimes mistake the inability to talk for indifference, the desire to be left alone, or for just being difficult and "not trying."

Family

Your first level of support will likely come from family. In some cases, a family member will become your Power of Attorney. Not because you are intellectually incapable of managing your care, but because you will need somebody to help communicate your wants and needs. A Power of Attorney is someone who legally acts on your behalf in financial, medical, or legal matters.

Be careful not to let your pride prevent family members from helping you. Speech-Language Pathologists encounter all types of family dynamics and people with aphasia tend to struggle with letting family manage some of their medical and financial affairs. It is important that your family member acknowledges that your intelligence is intact and that they review important decisions with you.

On the opposite spectrum, be aware of the condition of *learned helplessness.* Sometimes it is easy to give up and let someone else do everything for you just because they are willing. Make sure you continue doing things you are capable of even if it is a challenge and takes longer than usual. Letting someone else do things for you that you are capable of doing yourself will make the path to recovery much harder.

While the goal for recovery is as much independence as possible, it is also important to prioritize actives. Kim Huggins shares, "I know Christine can help load the dishwasher or help dust the house but it is more important for her to practice her conversation skills."

One of the many activities Kim does to help her daughter is to tell Christine at some time during the day, "It is your turn to talk and I will listen." Then Kim sits still and tries to respond with only gestures. She listens and waits patiently as Christine works to get the words out. She started small, and now three-and-a-half years later, they do this for 15–30 minutes a day. She adds, "It is our 'new normal'."

It is important for families to learn the skills needed to become an effective communication partner. Aphasia impacts you, but those you love as well. Communication affects so many aspects of your life and there is a lot of coping ahead for you and your family. It is not uncommon for there to be rough days for both you and your family. *Everyone* needs to adjust to this new life.

Aphasia recovery is not like breaking a bone and waiting for it to heal. Recovery will take a lot of work on your part and also from those who love you. There will be days you will not want to work hard. That is normal. One of the sayings Carol keeps on her desk is this: "Successful people do what needs to be done, whether they feel like it or not." The same is true for recovery. Being successful requires getting the job done even if you don't really feel like it. The choice is yours.

Often, the family is highly motivated and everyone wants you to push hard to recover. At the same time, everyone needs to be reminded that what you are going through is extremely difficult. Motivation will be naturally challenging.

Friends

Sadly, it is quite common for people to lose friends once they have aphasia. ARC members share that they have experienced some negative responses from others and sometimes find it difficult to retain their friends. Having strong supportive friendship patterns prior to aphasia can be helpful."[xxix]

When your friends come to visit you, let them know you are still the same person inside.

- I am the same inside but I am having trouble communicating.

It is unfortunate that people with aphasia are sometimes considered to be confused, mentally impaired, using drugs or alcohol, or have dementia. Not being able to answer orientation questions about the date and your location because of aphasia is much different than having dementia.

– *Slow down so I can process what you are saying.*

– *I am thinking but I have trouble speaking.*

Good friends are often eager to help you, but need to know what they can do to help. It might be uncomfortable for them at first to interact with you because you can't communicate the same way you could in the past. Have your friend help you with therapy goals, but most importantly enjoy your friendships and do things together.

Some activities that you might try later in your recovery may include: listening to music together, listening to an audio book, playing cards, and playing board games. Some games do not require much speaking, such as checkers, chess, bridge, poker, Rummikube®, Connect Four and Monopoly. Pick something that you enjoyed playing before your stroke or brain injury.

Other games are excellent for building communication skills but may be a challenge: Taboo, Catch Phrase, Charades, Pictionary, Scrabble®, Anomia, Scattergories, and Guess Who are all excellent choices as language-building games. Some of them may be quite difficult, but if you have a friend you feel comfortable with and is patient with you, it is definitely a great idea to try some of these games together. Ask your Speech-Language Pathologist for game suggestions based on your current abilities.

Aphasia can be isolating and lonely because of the inability to communicate. Friendship is extremely important. If your friend visits and isn't sure what you can do together, here are some things you can suggest:

- *Show me pictures on your smartphone*

- *Let's go out for coffee.*

- *Let's go out to lunch.*

- *Please bring a game for us to play.*

- *I'd like to go to a park and walk around.*

- *Let's go shopping together.*

- *Please bring your pet by for me to visit with.*

- *Let's watch a favorite movie.*

Connecting

The Aphasia Recovery Connection works to help connect people by offering opportunities for people with aphasia to meet. One husband of a person with aphasia shared, "I never heard my wife laugh after her stroke. One day I heard her laughing in another room. I went to check on her and saw her talking to Christine Huggins on a video call. They had met in Las Vegas at an ARC event. The two women were struggling to get their words out but there was a connection between them. It was so heart-warming to see my wife smiling again, even laughing."

When discussing the mission of our non-profit, the one word ARC continues to value the most is *connection*. David, Christine, and over one million others in the U.S. alone know the isolation aphasia brings. ARC works to bring people together, to find hope, share experiences, and help end the isolation for those who are recovering from aphasia.

Aphasia U Boot Camp

ARC is excited to be offering the Aphasia U Boot Camps. One of the major goals is to help connect people with aphasia as well as to offer family support.

The program starts with multiple workshops in Las Vegas and is then followed up with two to three weeks of daily interactions through video conferencing. We have lined up some of the top therapists in the country to present via video modules, including Dr. Audrey Holland, who is recognized worldwide for her aphasia work, and David's older brother, Dr. Mike Dow, a psychotherapist who frequently appears on *Dr. Oz* and *The Doctors* and who also serves on the Boot Camp Advisory Board. It is a new and exciting model as we are creating what we wish we had all along: fun, learning, hope, technology, sharing.

resources. options. goals. caring. Inspiration and most of all *connection*.

Building a Support Team

Carol was fortunate to have a strong support network when David had his stroke. Her good friend was a family therapist. In addition, her husband had endured a brain injury and never came home. He was living in a nursing home at the time of David's stroke. She gave Carol this valuable advice, "When people call and ask if there is anything they can do, your answer should be, 'Yes'." Most people with aphasia are in for a long road ahead and many life changes. It is a difficult time and it is best if you enlist the help of those who are willing.

You may be surprised by the amount of people in your life and in your community who are eager to help you. Do not be afraid or too proud to ask! You can use social media to reach out to your friends and family and ask for help. Your family members can reach out to your church, school, friends, family, and even local community centers to ask for volunteers to help you with your therapy goals. Not everyone can afford intensive therapy programs and you can enlist people in the community to help with your recovery.

Your therapist can provide the exercises and goals and your family can help coordinate volunteers to come help you with communication goals. Speech therapy sessions only make up a tiny percentage of your week. If you want to optimize recovery and are motivated, we suggest you find challenging and therapeutic activities to supplement your clinical therapy hours. You will learn more in the next chapter about some great options when we discuss technology.

Kim and Carol found it best to utilize volunteers to help with cooking, running errands, and doing other tasks while they work more intensively with their loved ones.

Maura Silverman M.S. CCC-SLP is the founder of Triangle Aphasia Project (TAP) in Raleigh, NC. This organization helps people with aphasia utilize their community to increase their rehabilitation potential. TAP provides guidelines for therapy and has volunteers help people maximize their recovery. They encourage people with aphasia to form a circle of support and reach out to their community to ask for help.

Maura encourages people with aphasia to remember that many people want to help with the recovery process, but are unsure of how to help. Engaging them in communication tasks will increase their understanding of aphasia, while helping the person with aphasia gain confidence to return to social, vocational, and recreational pursuits. A guided program allows for accessible language support and puts the ownership of the recovery process where it belongs, in the hands of the person with aphasia.

Maura is consulting with ARC for the Aphasia U Boot Camp Program. When scheduling a time to discuss Aphasia U Boot Camp, she mentioned she could meet with the ARC team *after* she trained a church 'family' to support a member of their congregation who has aphasia. That is a perfect example of how Life Participation Approach to Aphasia works. Support people where they live and help them build a support system for success!

Aphasia Recovery Connection offers many videos and opportunities online for others to learn more about aphasia. Many friends and families of those with aphasia also share their experiences and challenges on Facebook which is a way to learn from others who are walking in your shoes. There is no 'right' or 'wrong' way to approach things; what is important is to base the choices on the person with aphasia and your own family dynamics.

Support Groups

Aphasia Recovery Connection is an award-winning resource that offers connections through Facebook for meeting others as you work on recovery. Even if you have never joined Facebook before, it is worth joining for the benefits ARC offers. Once you join the group, you will have access to thousands of other individuals who are facing similar challenges. Knowing you are not alone in your struggle can be quite powerful and healing.

ARC provides support and offers a place to share with people that deal with the same challenges and experiences you are having. ARC also posts questions and videos to help members with aphasia practice reading, writing, and comprehension. We even hold annual live events including cruises and excursions so you and your family can socialize and learn from others who have been impacted by aphasia. On the cruises, we also have speakers who discuss topics about aphasia.

The National Stroke Association awarded the Aphasia Recovery Connection a RAISE Award for making an positive impact on stroke survivors. It is an honor to help connect people. Connection is powerful, especially for people who may have lost jobs or friends as they deal with this devastating and often misunderstood disability.

The National Aphasia Association (NAA) is another good resource for support. They provide a variety of information about aphasia for both people with the condition as well as their caregivers. **aphasia.org/naa-network** helps you search for local support groups around the United States. These local support groups provide an opportunity to increase communication skills and share with others. They are often led by a Speech-Language Pathologist.

Support groups are a great way to increase the amount of time you socialize and challenge yourself. Support groups can provide emotional reinforcement by simply letting you share and hear others' stories. In these safe settings, remember to challenge yourself and talk, even if you know you are going to make mistakes.

Communication Groups

The American Speech-Language-Hearing Association (ASHA) is another valuable resource for individuals with aphasia. You can visit **asha.org** to find a local graduate or undergraduate speech therapy program near you. Look for "Find an Education Program" on their site. Most graduate programs offer clinics to the public at a very low cost. Even if you are currently in therapy, take advantage of the extra therapy and sign up. Often it is hard for graduate programs to find enough adults for their students' clinical hours. They will be happy to have the opportunity to work with you. In fact, that is how David Dow and Amanda Anderson met over ten years ago, as patient and graduate student clinician.

If there isn't a graduate program near your home, recruit local high school students who are looking for volunteer hours. Four years after his stroke, I was able to find someone to work with David by calling a local Catholic school that required volunteer hours. The student was grateful for the opportunity to work with David and was glad to add the experience to his college application. They worked together with aphasia workbooks, reading, and played games. David's therapist assisted with the selection of materials which ensured they were working at levels that were appropriate for David.

Staying Active

As you recover, volunteering to help others can be quite beneficial. Despite your aphasia, you still have a great deal to offer. Staying active and having a passion for something is extremely important. Look for opportunities to volunteer, join new groups, stay active in past hobbies or start new ones. Everybody needs goals and something to keep busy and the therapeutic benefits are huge. The worst possible thing you can do is isolate yourself, cut off interaction with the world and stay on the couch watching TV. There is an active world of people with aphasia. ARC provides the opportunity to reach out to them, make new friends and become involved.

Avi Golden is a stroke survivor with aphasia who exemplifies the qualities of someone who refuses to give up and continues to stay active. Staying active and continuing to challenge yourself is key to successful rehabilitation and overcoming the challenges of life post-stroke. Before his stroke, Avi was a paramedic and about to start medical school. Avi loved many different outdoor sports like horseback riding, kayaking, sailing, bicycle riding and snowboarding.

When Avi was 33, he had a massive stroke that weakened his right side and resulted in aphasia. Avi didn't let his stroke hold him back. He started a group called New York Outdoor Disability that helps people with disabilities participate in outdoor sports. He also continues to volunteer as a paramedic and participates in a variety of plays. He advocates for people with aphasia and stays as involved as possible. Inside, he is still the same driven and smart individual and he hasn't let his stroke change who he is.

Adjusting to life with aphasia is challenging. You will have many hurdles to overcome. It will be frustrating when people assume that you are not intelligent just because you struggle to communicate. Make goals for yourself to stay active. Volunteer, get outside, exercise, call friends and try to continue doing things you love to do. Therapy doesn't have to be the only opportunity you have to improve your language function. Life itself provides endless challenges of real world situations to improve your skills.

**1995. David Dow's brain scan.
David could not read, write, or speak.**

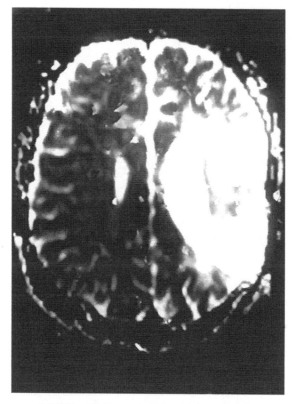

NEU•RO•PLAS•TIC•I•TY

Neuroplasticity is the brain's ability to adapt and
maximize remaining functions after a brain injury.

*The image is David looking down. The brain damage is on *his* left side.

Chapter 5

Neuroplasticity

Aphasia is a result of damaged brain cells in the language center of your brain. The left hemisphere typically is the dominant hemisphere for both language comprehension and production. Broca's area, located in the left frontal lobe of the brain, controls language production while Wernicke's area lies on the left posterior temporal lobe of the brain and controls language comprehension. All strokes, no matter what kind, damage brain cells. The size and location of the lesion caused by your stroke or brain injury will determine what type of aphasia you have.

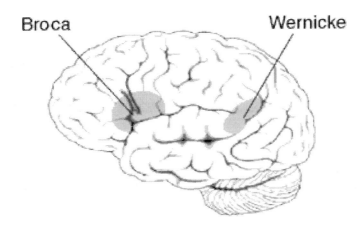

xxx

Language is a series of messages sent throughout the brain from one neuron to the next. When overcoming trauma, the human brain is remarkable and has the capability to reorganize areas of the brain and can even switch language centers from one hemisphere of the brain to the other. The brain can also build new neural connections to repair damaged areas. This phenomenon is called neuroplasticity. Basically, the brain has the ability to repair and build new neural pathways after a stroke or brain injury which has damaged brain cells.

Christine Huggins explains, "Your brain is moving every second and your neurons are wiring different things. Speech therapy, 'tweaks' (your brain) in different paths. It is really exhausting. It's like a big workout for your brain."

After a stroke or brain injury, the brain is able to repair itself at the neural level by growing new neural connections. New neural pathways are formed when one axon grows new nerve endings to reconnect neurons that were severed as a result of damage from a stroke or brain injury.[xxxi] In other words, new neural pathways are formed to reconnect areas of the brain. Because of neuroplasticity, continued recovery of both physical and language function is possible through rehabilitation.

How to Facilitate Neuroplasticity

You just suffered a stroke or brain injury, and from your perspective there isn't anything positive about that, but in the world of rehabilitation, strokes and brain injury recovery can be very promising. Neuroplasticity makes recovery possible. It will not be easy. It can take years and a network of support to get back many lost skills. Unlike progressive diseases like Parkinson's, Multiple Sclerosis or ALS, stroke survivors have the potential to improve.

Neurogenesis is the growth of new brain cells and makes recovery of language and physical function possible.[xxxii] There are things you can do to help facilitate neurogenesis. When you wake up every morning remind yourself, "My brain is repairing itself." Use every resource available to help your brain recover and regain function.

Preventing Strokes

Things you can do to reduce the risk of additional strokes are eat healthy and exercise. There is a wealth of information available how to reduce your risk of stroke. The American Heart Association has an interactive risk factor assessment tool on their website:

mylifecheck.heart.org

The National Stroke Association also has information on their website regarding what stroke risk factors you can control, such as high blood pressure, smoking, diabetes, carotid and other artery disease, atrial fibrillation, high cholesterol, physical inactivity, obesity, excessive alcohol consumption, and illegal drug use, and how to curtail the risks.[xxxiii]

It is important that you understand what you can do to reduce your risk of stroke. For example, according to the American Heart Association, smoking nearly doubles your risk of ischemic stroke. [xxxiv]

Fortunately, the American Heart Association reports rapid decreases in mortality rates and incidents of ischemic strokes with the immediate cessation of smoking.[xxxv] The National Stroke Association reports that within 5 years of the first stroke, the chance of having a recurrent stroke increases as much as 40%.[xxxvi] Second strokes have higher death rates and more severe disabilities since part of the brain has already been injured and is not as resilient to trauma. [xxxvii] Become your own advocate and get proactive about your health. Find out why you had your first stroke and do everything you can to reduce your risk of having another.

If you have another stroke, knowing the symptoms and acting immediately can save your life. The National Stroke Association promotes a way to help remember the signs and symptoms of stroke:

FAST:

Face: Look in the mirror and smile or have someone check to see if one side of your face is drooping.

Arm: Raise both of your arms, does one droop downwards? Does one arm feel numb or tingle?

Speech: Try to say a simple sentence. Are you able to get the words out? Is your speech slurred? Does your tongue feel numb?

Time: If you present with these symptoms, call 911 immediately to receive the proper care to prevent further damage to your brain.[xxxviii]

How Rehabilitation Works

We know that the brain has the capability to rewire itself through the power of neuroplasticity. This doesn't happen overnight and a balance of patient motivation, strong community support and rehabilitation all come together to make continued recovery possible. How exactly do external forces and stimulus cause the brain to begin to change and language begin to improve?

Strokes can cause hemiparesis or weakness on one side of the body. With aphasia the brain has difficulty with word retrieval and sometimes speech can be slurred (dysarthria) or have motor planning difficulties (apraxia). Remember that with all of these impairments, initially the muscles and nerves in the legs, arms, tongue and face have not been directly damaged. The brain is where the damage occurred. By moving the impaired area with assistance of a therapist and using muscles surrounding the weakened area, you can stimulate the brain near the damaged area. This stimulation can promote neurogenesis.

Research studies have shown that even micro exercises, such as moving your thumb back and forth for 15 minutes, can cause the brain to form new neural connections.[xxxix] Aphasia is unique to stroke impairments because there isn't any visible impairment. The neural pathways for word retrieval in the language center of the brain have been damaged. To translate the concept of small exercises for aphasia try repeating communication activities throughout the day that are easy for you. Ask your speech therapist for suggestions.

It is important not to rely solely on speech therapy sessions to improve. even if you have speech therapy 5 times a week for an hour each time, that is less than 3% of the week that you spend in speech therapy.

Repetition is essential to improving both motor function and language function.[xl] You will want to start doing some of the exercises that you do in therapy during the day and make it part of your daily routine. Start by trying to say aloud what you do throughout the day. Name items around your room as you use them. After a commercial on TV, say the name of the product that is for sale. Narrate what you do as you do it. "I'm picking up my hair brush. I'm moving it from the top of my head to the back of my head." Even if you are only able to get a few of the words out, it is the attempt that matters because it stimulates the brain to begin the formation of new neural pathways.

Research studies also show that challenging activities help the recovery of language function. Physical therapists utilize constraint induced movement therapy for stroke survivors. This strategy constrains the unaffected arm of a stroke survivor with hemiparesis, having them use the arm that had been weakened by the stroke.[xli] The weak limb is isolated to complete daily tasks and tackle exercises which produced great results in rehabilitation. This same concept has been carried over into language therapy for aphasia.

Studies have reproduced constraint induced therapy for aphasia. When somebody with aphasia uses the mode of communication that takes the least amount of effort, it is considered similar to using their unaffected arm or leg in physical therapy.[xlii] It is human nature to avoid frustration and take the path of least resistance. In aphasia rehabilitation, the more communication challenges that are taken on in everyday situations, the better the chances are for a fuller recovery.[xliii]

Constraint induced therapy that incorporates gradual steps up to difficult tasks has been shown to have excellent results for individuals who were told they had already reached their maximum post-stroke potential.[xliv] The basis of constraint induced therapy for aphasia is to incorporate the most difficult communication tasks into therapy and everyday life, regardless of frustration level, to achieve the highest levels of expressive language communication abilities.

You would be hard-pressed to find any research that showed that less interaction and communication translated into better recovery for somebody with aphasia. The most important thing you can do for yourself is to stay active and communicate as much as possible.

Challenge yourself and even if something is frustrating, remember that a frustrating task is one that promotes the formation of new neural pathways. David, states in his book, Brain Attack, "Stroke survivors need to fight for recovery with determination and hope. It takes a long time to recover."

There are many resources available to help carry over therapy activities and make recovery part of your life, not just the hour or so you spend in speech therapy every week. To be successful, you need to find ways to challenge yourself throughout the day, every day. Motivation, family and community support, social interaction, and determination to challenge yourself to get better is the perfect combination for a strong recovery.

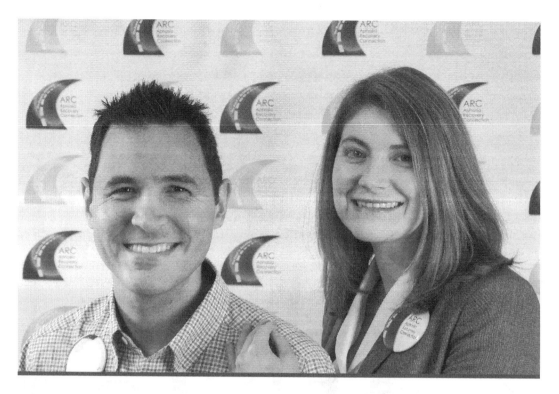

APHASIA RECOVERY CONNECTION
FOUNDERS & STROKE SURVIVORS

We have aphasia. It affects many things. Things are not as easy as before, but we are working hard to adapt, cope, and improve. We are also working hard on Aphasia Recovery.

We will not stop trying. It takes determination and persistence to fight for recovery. Keep trying.

Christine Huggins & David Dow

Chapter 6

Types of Aphasia Therapy

Since no two cases of aphasia are exactly the same, there are many types of speech therapy approaches. Therapy builds on neuroplasticity by starting with language tasks that you are able to do and gradually increasing the difficulty level to improve your ability with harder tasks. This chapter will explain the common types of speech therapy techniques for aphasia. Your Speech-Language Pathologist can individualize your treatment and focus on goals that are the most important to you.

Aphasia Treatments

ASHA has recognized the therapies described in this chapter as potential treatments for aphasia. It is unlikely your therapist will use just one type of treatment. Ideally, your therapy will combine a variety of these approaches.[xlv] It will be helpful to know what types of therapy are available.

Computer Based Therapy

Computer software programs for aphasia allow for specific training on a language deficit. Computer based treatments are helpful to track progress and demonstrate improvement. Some of the benefits of computer based therapy include: flexibility, repetition, and the ability to personalize language exercises.[xlvi] There are many options to choose from if you are looking for a computer based program to use. AphasiaSoftwareFinder.org provides a helpful list of available aphasia software. Outpatient therapy clinics are more likely to have aphasia focused software available for patients to use. You can tell your speech therapist:

- *I'd like to try a computer software program for aphasia*
- *What programs do you have?*
- *What programs do you recommend?*

You can post a question on the ARC Facebook group site to see what programs members with aphasia like.

Constraint Induced Language Therapy (CILT)

Constraint induced language therapy, or CILT, is based on the concept that if you force yourself to use the mode of communication that is the hardest, you will make the most progress. CILT is typically an intensive program of up to 3 hours a day, 5 days a week. Your speech therapist will help with cues to initiate speech during communication tasks. CILT discourages use of aphasia compensatory strategies such as gestures or writing and focuses solely on verbal responses. CILT takes advantage of neuroplasticity to structure tasks that facilitate the formation of new neural connections in the language centers of the brain.

Melodic Intonation Therapy

Melodic Intonation Therapy (MIT) utilizes rhythm and melody to improve expressive language function. The right hemisphere of the brain controls our ability to listen to and produce music. Most people who have aphasia have sustained damage to the left hemisphere of the brain. Melodic Intonation Therapy recruits the right hemisphere using music to help with language tasks.

MIT therapy is usually presented in four stages. In the first stage, the therapist and patient will hum a phrase from a familiar song. For the second phrase, the patient and therapist will sing the words together. Next, the person with aphasia will sing the phrase independently. In the fourth and final stage, the person with aphasia may be able to speak the phrase.[xlvii] Finger tapping is also utilized to help facilitate rhythmic speech and recruit additional regions of the brain to help with expressive language. [xlviii] During Melodic Intonation Therapy, SLPs sometimes incorporate melody into conversations and have a person with aphasia participate in a conversation by singing the answers to questions.

Christine shared that she also enjoyed music while in the hospital, recalling that a music therapist brought his guitar and sang familiar songs. Kim, her mom, said that as Christine's body swayed with the music, a few sounds escaped from her mouth. "It warmed my heart," she shared.

Word Finding Treatment

Word finding difficulty, or anomia, is one of the hallmark symptoms of aphasia. Most types of aphasia have some degree of anomia associated with it. Speech-Language Pathologists will use cues to help a person with aphasia say a specific word.

Semantic cues are verbal prompts related to the meaning of the word. For example, if you are trying to say *bed*, your SLP would cue you by saying "sleep", "lie down in it", or "king-sized."

Your SLP can also help you using phonemic cues which are the initial sounds of the word you want to say. For example, if you are trying to name a photograph of a shoe, your SLP would make the sound "sh" to help you retrieve the word.

Gesture cues are also helpful with word finding tasks. Using your hand to pretend to use an object, triggers other areas of your brain to help retrieve the desired word. Your SLP may also use carrier phrases to decrease anomia. If you are stuck on the word "dog", the prompt "It's raining cats and _____" may help you say *dog*.

Multimodal Treatment

Multimodal treatment focuses on using alternative modes of communication. Augmentative and Alternative Communication (AAC) is an example of an alternative mode of communication. AAC devices can be basic picture images on a communication board or a complex computer device designed to help an individual with aphasia communicate. Your SLP can help you pick an AAC device that best suits your needs. DynoVox and Lingraphia are two companies that make specialized AAC devices for individuals with aphasia. There is also software available for your tablet that can function as an AAC device. Individuals with very limited expressive language function can benefit greatly from using an AAC device. You can tell your speech therapist:

- *I am interested in trying an AAC device*

Visual Action Therapy

Visual Action Therapy is a treatment approach used with individuals with global aphasia. This approach teaches individuals with global aphasia to communicate using hand and arm gestures.[xlix] The Visual Action Therapy treatment approach is appropriate for people with severe expressive and comprehension deficits. Visual Action Therapy uses real objects, line drawings of objects and pictures of people using objects. This therapy approach combines pointing to items and gesturing the function of objects to improve expressive and receptive language skills.[l]

Promoting Aphasia Communication Effectiveness (PACE)

This type of therapy can be tried at home. You will need photographs of functional objects or index cards with the names of objects written on them. As the items become easier for you, try using verbs or picture scenes.

For this type of exercise, select a photograph of an item and then you and a partner will take turns trying to guess what the photo is. It is similar to the game "20 questions" but instead of asking and answering yes or no questions, ask questions that require a description for an answer. Questions such as "Where can you find it?", "What do you use it for?", "Who uses it?" and "When do you use it?" are ideal because they require a descriptive answer. PACE encourages a person with aphasia to communicate any way possible by drawing, writing, gesturing, and describing.[li]

Oral Reading for Language in Aphasia (ORLA)

ORLA techniques have the person with aphasia read sentences aloud, first in unison with a partner and then independently. Try pacing yourself with your finger as you point to each word and keep a steady rhythm as you read. Repeating the same sentences several times is recommended. As you improve, you can move on to reading paragraphs and passages aloud. Research has shown that practicing reading aloud with a partner and then reading aloud independently can carry over to improved expressive language skills.[lii]

Partner Approaches

Partner approaches have the Speech-Language Pathologist work together with the person with aphasia and somebody they have the most interaction with, such as a spouse or children. Conversational Coaching Therapy concentrates on communication between you and your most frequent conversational partner. Supported Communication Intervention therapy involves an SLP helping a person with aphasia and a family member communicate together.

Speech Therapy for aphasia can be highly individualized. You can work on communication goals that are most important to you. Some people with aphasia are able to have a conversation with their SLP after they have worked together, but they continue to struggle when they try to speak to family members. You can also have your speech therapist work with you and your family member so you can practice communication goals at home. You can add talking with your spouse or family member to your speech therapy goals. Say:

- *I want to practice communicating with my spouse/family/friend.*
- *Please show my family member how to work on my therapy goals with me.*

Life Participation Approach

Life Participation Approach concentrates on real life communication goals as a part of therapy. The focus of Life Participation Approach is to help a person with aphasia participate in communication situations where they may need support. Goals are made based on community interaction and the level of support an individual needs to participate in desired activities. Therapy can focus on overcoming communication obstacles by treating both the person with aphasia and the people they interact with the most.

Life Participation Approach is a model of therapy that embraces goals to reduce barriers in day-to-day communication. Types of goals for this approach range from communicating with family to challenges associated with returning to work, depending on which area requires the most focus.

Speech-Language Pathologists work to make a person's environment more "aphasia-friendly." This model of therapy not only focuses on the person with aphasia but others who are indirectly affected by aphasia, like family members, friends, colleagues, and service providers. It is a patient-centered philosophy that gives priority to real life situations.

The ARC Aphasia U Boot Camp is based on the Life Participation Approach to Aphasia. With today's limited insurance options for people with aphasia, we realize that people with aphasia need a new option that engages them educationally and socially to utilize their skills and learn new ones. Often, when we do an ARC event, we see people with aphasia teaching one another. They have a wealth of information to share with one another!

We have been consulting with many of the nation's top Speech-Language Pathologists to design a breakthrough program. People with aphasia need something that is fun, but that also works! It is a program that is affordable and builds connection. The Aphasia U Boot Camp will launch in the Fall of 2015. Space will be limited to keep the group size small and produce the best results. If you would like more information, email us at ARCaphasia@gmail.com

Aphasia U Boot Camp aims to empower people with aphasia to take therapy into their own hands. You will learn how to incorporate language building activities into your everyday life. Most importantly, Aphasia U Boot Camp will help people with aphasia build connections. Meeting others with aphasia who you are comfortable talking with can be life changing. ARC's mission to end isolation for people with aphasia will be the heart and soul of Aphasia U Boot Camp.

Aphasia U Boot Camp has the support of some of the top aphasia experts in the country. Carol shares, " We are so excited to team up with such great experts. This program will be like no other and we are designing exactly what David, Christine and people with aphasia have been telling us they want and need. ARC is going to deliver!"

The American Stroke Association provides a list of aphasia centers that embrace the Life Participation Approach for Aphasia.

Life Participation Approach Centers

Alder Aphasia Center Maywood New Jersey 201- 368- 8585

Aphasia Center of California Oakland California 510 -336- 0112

Aphasia Center of Tucson. Tuscon, Arizona 520- 730- 8428

Aphasia Center of West Texas Midland, Texas 432 - 699- 1261

Aphasia Communication Enhancement Program Kalamazoo,MI 269-387-7000

Aphasia Institute Toronto, Ontario, Canada 416-226-3636 ext 24

Aphasia Resource Center Boston University 617-353-0197

Communication Recovery Groups at St. Jude Fullerton, CA 714-992-3000

Communication Recovery Groups at CSU Sacramento, California 916-278-6695

Dalhousie Aphasia Clinic Halifax, Nova Scotia 902-494-5158

Houston Aphasia Recovery Center Houston, TX 713-781-7100

Moss Rehab Aphasia Center Philadelphia, PA 215-663-6554

RIC for Aphasia Research and Treatment Chicago, Illinois 312-238-6163

Snyder Center for Aphasia Life Enhancement Baltimore 410-323-1777

Stroke Comeback Center Vienna, Virginia 703-255-5221

The Aphasia House Orlando 407-882-0468

Triangle Aphasia Project Unlimited Raleigh, NC 919-650-3854

Script Training

Script Training is a type of therapy that you can try at home. Scripts can be used with many types of aphasia and are most successful when they are practiced over and over. Repetition of a script leads to carryover of communication skills. Your SLP can help create a script you can practice at home with a partner. Pick something you are interested in and something that is a real life situation such as: calling to order a pizza, making a doctor's appointment, talking about the birth of a child or a favorite vacation destination. Dr. Audrey Holland notes that for a script to be successful, it has to be fun and personally meaningful. Ideal scripts are about 8 to 15 sentences long and have around 8 turn-taking sets.[liii]

Scripts can be monologues where somebody is the only speaker or dialogues which require a partner to ask and answer questions. First try easier scripts such as, "Hello. My name is ___. I had a stroke." Then progress to longer dialogue scripts. You should practice reading the script over and over until you have memorized it and do not need the written cues. Make scripts that are real life situations.

You can ask your Speech-Language Pathologist:

Please help me make more scripts that I can practice at home.

Dialogue Script:
Script: Ordering a Pizza

- Thanks for calling Pappy's Pizza. Can I help you?

- Yes, I'd like to order a large pizza.

- Would you like any toppings?

- Yes, pepperoni and sausage.

- Would you like any side items?

- Yes, I'd like an order of breadsticks with extra dipping sauce.

- Anything else?

- Yes, I'd like a 2 liter bottle of Sprite

- What is your address?

- (Say your address)

- What time would you like the pizza delivered?

- Right away please.

- How would you like to pay?

- Cash.

- Thank you for your order. It should arrive in 45 minutes.

- Great! Thank you.

Other Aphasia Treatments

Some people with aphasia have difficulty with specific language tasks. There are specialized aphasia therapy programs to isolate the area where a person with aphasia is having trouble. For example, Reading Treatment, Writing Treatment, Syntax Treatment, Treatment of Underlying Forms and Verb Network Strengthening Treatment are all specialized aphasia therapy techniques.[liv] To read more about these specific therapies and evidence based research showing the data from clinical studies, visit: **asha.org**

Remember that *you* are in charge of your rehabilitation. If you feel that you want to vary the challenge or make a change with a new speech therapist, it is up to you to voice these goals and desires. Sometimes, a change is fresh and exciting and we all tend to get bored if there are no changes in our lives.

Unless you are participating in a clinical research trial, it is unlikely you will only use only one of these aphasia therapy techniques. Your SLP will use a combination of these techniques to best meet your needs. If you continue to do the same exercises over and over, and you haven't seen any improvement outside of therapy, it is okay to ask your SLP to modify your treatment plan.

You can ask your SLP:

- *Can we try another approach to therapy?*

- *I am interested in including my family in therapy.*

- *I'm getting frustrated with our current exercises, can we try something else?*

- *I feel successful when I read aloud. Can we work that into therapy?*

- *I would like to practice using my tablet apps in therapy.*

- *I would like to give Melodic Intonation Therapy a try.*

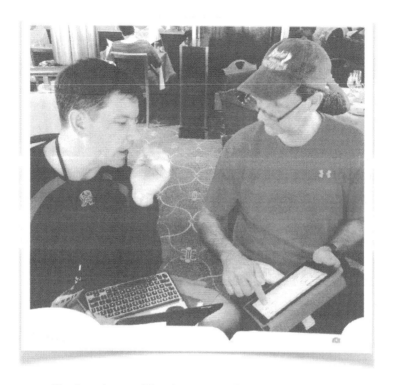

Technology, Sharing, and Communicating

Chris and Rob are both stroke survivors who were working as engineers prior to their strokes. Here, they are sharing iPad apps with one another.

They met on an ARC Aphasia cruise. It is helpful for people to share ideas, experiences, and challenges. Often, friendships form and aphasia is not as lonely.

They utilize technology to help communicate. The iPad has been a big help to them. Both use a white board app so they can write down key words.

Chapter 7

Technology for Aphasia

In this age of tablets and smartphones, there are many helpful programs for aphasia. Technology can be utilized for assisting with communication. Speech therapy computer software or tablet applications for aphasia can be used on your own or with a Speech-Language Pathologist. Incorporating technology into your rehabilitation is also a helpful way to maximize your recovery potential.

Tablets

If you used a tablet before aphasia, continue to use what you are familiar with. If you've never used a tablet before, it may be worth the investment to purchase one. Most SLPs would recommend purchasing an iPad, to have access to the widest variety of programs (or *apps,* as they're often called.) To save money, you could purchase a used or refurbished iPad, but make sure that it is compatible with the latest software you plan on using for your rehabilitation.

Kindle devices are quite affordable and have many options for aphasia apps. You can search for 'aphasia' apps on the amazon website. Search aphasia and click the arrow next to the search bar to select apps for Androids. This will show you what is available. You can ask ARC members for feedback about a particular app or tablet preferences.

If you do not have access to a computer, getting a tablet will function as both a device that can access the internet, an Augmentative Alternative Communication (AAC) device and provide access to apps for speech therapy exercises.

Christine's stroke was in 2011. A friend stopped by for a visit three months after her stroke and offered to loan her an iPad. Her mom shares, "We immediately bought aphasia apps, many of them were only 99 cents. We also bought some preschool apps.

I remember one Christine used for several weeks called *Photo Touch* by Grasshopper. Four photos appeared on the iPad screen, such as a cat, dog, ball, and a cup. A voice would say, 'touch the ball,' and she would follow the direction given. If correct, the box would light up. Sometimes, it would take over ten seconds before selecting an answer. Sometimes, she would repeat the questions several times. It took incredible effort for her to process just one word."

She has progressed a lot since then. In fact, David and Christine are speaking to speech therapists at their national convention in 2014 to share how technology apps helped supplement their therapy or helped them when therapy ran out.

Facebook

Aphasia Recovery Connection has a private Facebook group and a public page that are great resources and offer peer support within a virtual community. ARC members on Facebook enjoy having a place where they can communicate and practice their skills such as reading, writing and posting videos. ARC's Facebook group also offers the opportunity to receive support as well as socializing with other people with aphasia.

If you haven't joined the ARC Facebook group yet, now is the time! Appendix C explains how to create a Facebook account. Once you have an account, search in the top search box for the Aphasia Recovery Connection group. After you click on the group, its main page will come up. Under the photograph on the right side, click *Join*. It will take a little while for the group's administrators to approve your request. Once you have joined, you will be able to comment and post questions. Since it is a closed group, your Facebook friends will not see your questions or comments.

There are multiple groups on Facebook that are beneficial for stroke survivors. ARC has groups for caregivers and friends. There are groups for young stroke survivors and their family members. Facebook can be a wonderful resource to find support from others who are dealing with similar issues. The Speech Therapy Aphasia Rehabilitation (STAR) group on Facebook provides free therapy exercises for people with aphasia.

APPS

An app (short for application) is something you can download onto either a smartphone or tablet like an iPad or Kindle device. There are many free apps that you can use on your mobile device of choice.

If you search for "flash cards", lots of free options with many naming categories will come up. You can use basic flash cards to work on word retrieval skills. Try to select one where you can mute the word. It might be helpful at first to have the app say the name of the object with you initially and, as you improve, you can mute the word. You can also search for "aphasia" for apps with more appropriate exercises.

The app "Heads Up" that Ellen Degeneres plays on her show requires you to describe the word that somebody holds up above their head, and they have to guess what it is. This is an excellent game to work on descriptive language skills that promotes the formation of new neural pathways. "Heads Up" also comes in a board game edition. ARC hosts video chats about new and helpful apps for aphasia. Some apps that we have recently recommended are:

Asking TherAppy	**Pictello (scripts)**
Locabulary Lite	**Small Talk (scripts)**
Word Stack	**Oxford Picture Dictionary**
Chain of Thought	**Taboo**
Constant Therapy	**Just Say It**
Tactus Therapy Apps	**Words with Friends**
Alicom	**iConverse (scripts)**
Sonoflex Lite	**Make Change**
White Board	**Dollar and Cents**

Some of the apps are free and some of them cost a few dollars. Therapy applications and software with a wide variety of exercises and goals can cost somewhat more. Keep in mind that some of those apps are excellent products and they often cost less than a speech therapy session if you were to pay out of pocket.

On **aphasiarecoveryconnection.org** you can find

recommendations for current technology to help you communicate.

ARC has no affiliation with any technology companies and only

recommends products they think can benefit members. Several other

websites list apps and software for aphasia. Some of the ones that ARC

has found helpful are:

AphasiaSoftwareFinder.org

janefarrall.com/aac

tactustherapy.com/adultapplist.pdf

amyspeechlanguagetherapy.com/communication-boards.html

AAC

Before smartphones and tablets, Augmentative and Alternative

Communication (AAC) devices were bulky and cumbersome. Now

there are apps that you can download onto a device like an iPhone or

iPad and use it to help you communicate. Earlier AAC devices stuck

out and drew attention to the user. Today, almost everyone carries a

smartphone or tablet and it isn't unusual to see somebody using one.

Companies such as Lingraphica make a variety of AAC devices.

These are handheld speech-generating devices. They also provide a

variety of apps for speech therapy exercises as well as AAC on the go.

Their website, aphasia.com, offers a wealth of information about their products and how to get help with funding.

Some apps function as AAC devices. The app *YesNo* provides two buttons for yes/no that you can customize with your own voice. The apps *Scene Speak*, and *Scene and Heard* are communication boards with voice output. There are apps that function as complete AAC devices such as *MyVoice*, *Proloquo2Go* and *TalkTablet*. The full-functioning AAC apps range in price from $80 to around $200.[lv]

Software

Software is similar to an app and can even be the same program, but it is something that you use on your computer or laptop. There is software available for people with aphasia. Bungalow Software is one of multiple companies that make a variety of programs for aphasia. The Rehabilitation Institute of Chicago has aphasia script software programs using the script therapy technique. To view their software product go to: **ricaphasiascripts.contentshelf.com**

AphasiaSoftwareFinder.org has a nice aphasia-friendly list of aphasia software with a comparison table. Software programs can be an excellent way to supplement therapy and to continue speech therapy, especially near the end of the year when your speech therapy insurance benefits have been exhausted.

eWriters

For people with aphasia who have strong writing skills or who need written cues to improve comprehension, an eWriter is an excellent option. eWriters are inexpensive (under $50) electronic notepads that you can clear with the touch of a button. Some models allow you to save your image. An eWriter doesn't require paper and pencils and the stylus (pen) clips onto the board, making it aphasia-friendly. This is a nice device to aid with communication for people with aphasia. One of the most widely available is called the Boogie Board and available at places like Walmart or Amazon.

Other Technology

Kindle books are ones that you can read on a computer, smartphone, or tablet. You can hold multiple books on your tablet, which is aphasia-friendly, especially for people with right hand weakness. You can change the font size with digital books, which can help improve comprehension for some people with aphasia. Kindle books are relatively inexpensive compared to printed versions. You can also purchase aphasia workbooks for Kindle such as the first expressive language *Speech Therapy Aphasia Rehabilitation STAR Workbook.*

You can take advantage of tools that automatically come with your smartphone or tablet. The voice dictation on your smartphone can be a useful exercise. Turn it on and try reading or saying a sentence in a very clear rhythmic style. These voice dictation programs have difficulty perfectly recognizing what people without aphasia say, so it is sometimes quite a challenge, but will force you to speak in a slow rhythmic tone, which can help with expressive language function.

Phone conversations can be difficult for someone with aphasia. The programs Skype or ooVoo are ways to make video calls. Video calls can help people with aphasia communicate much better over long distances. Video chats allow for the use of facial expressions, gestures, photographs, and nods to help you communicate much better with people than you could over the telephone.

Technology and Therapy

If working on a computer or tablet is difficult for you, it is a perfect goal for speech therapy or occupational therapy. OTs can focus on some of the fine motor challenges involved in manipulating a tablet or computer. Working with technology is a wonderful skill that will help you with your communication. Tell your therapist.

- *I'd like to make working on my tablet a goal for therapy.*

- *I want to learn how to use Facebook in therapy.*

- *I'd like to practice writing emails in therapy.*

- *I'd like learn how to post a question on the ARC website.*

- *I would like to practice making a video call.*

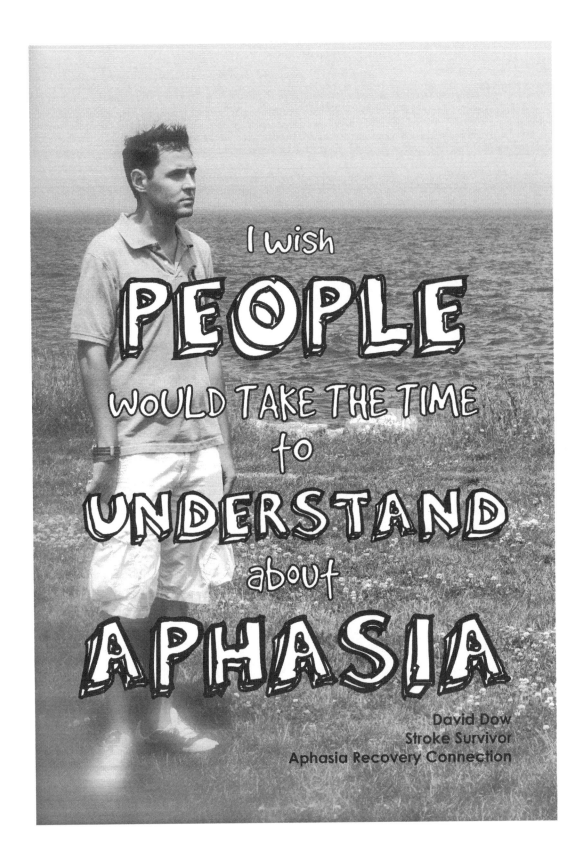

I wish PEOPLE WOULD TAKE THE TIME to UNDERSTAND about APHASIA

David Dow
Stroke Survivor
Aphasia Recovery Connection

Chapter 8

Coping

Nobody plans on having aphasia. It isn't something you can just ignore and then move on with your life. Aphasia can cause upheaval in every aspect of your life from career to relationships. You are not alone. Over a million people in the United States have aphasia. ARC is passionate about helping people touched by aphasia learn to cope and eventually thrive.

It is okay to cry, scream, and get angry! You didn't ask for this and you certainly do not deserve it. Aphasia is extremely frustrating and sadly, it is hard to find people, even health professionals, who are well versed in aphasia. People living with aphasia will tell you that having a support network like ARC can make all the difference in the world. Hope and motivation are your friends, isolation and despair your enemies. Even so, it is still okay to cry.

Carol Dow-Richards shares, "I know this is difficult. I lived this nightmare myself and know the feeling of being so very afraid and full of grief as a caregiver. I can only imagine how difficult it is for you. I know it is hard...and you must hang on to hope. Things do improve. However, it is often a very slow process."

Aphasia can be one of the most difficult deficits to cope with because of the lack of ability to communicate. Communication is how we vent, how we feel better. When you get in a fight, you talk things out to make amends. When you are afraid, you talk about what is bothering you. When you are depressed, you talk to somebody about what is weighing on you. Aphasia robs you of these outlets.

Depression

As many as 62% of people with aphasia are clinically depressed one year after their stroke.[lvi] Up to 33% of people with aphasia have major depression, at the one year mark after their initial diagnosis.[lvii] Stroke survivors can experience major depression which results from a chemical imbalance in the brain.[lviii] A psychiatrist can evaluate you and determine if you would benefit from antidepressant medication. Stroke and brain injury survivors also experience Reactive Depression.[lix] Reactive Depression results from a life-altering event. Ask yourself: *Would I be depressed if I didn't have aphasia?*

People with aphasia experience a great loss of their former abilities and go through a period of grief.[lx] It is understandable to mourn. There is some controversy whether or not people experiencing grief go through set standard stages.[lxi] Remember, your journey of

acceptance and coping is as unique as you and your aphasia.[lxii]

David Dow shares with ARC members a tip to stay positive: "I

know it is very difficult to be motivated and active during your

recovery. One of my sayings is *don't be a couch potato.* It is very easy

for me and many people to sit on the couch and watch TV and not care

about the world around you. I think it is very important to get out there

and keep moving and keep your brain active every day."

Emotional Lability

Stroke and brain injury survivors may experience unexpected and

exaggerated changes in mood which is called emotional lability. You

may find yourself crying for no apparent reason or laughing

uncontrollably. Your stroke or brain injury may have damaged the part

of your brain that regulates and controls emotions.[lxiii] It is important for

family and friends to understand.

Changes in mood may result in increased irritability, anger or

intense sadness. Sometimes the strong emotions such as crying or

laughing are not related to how you are feeling inside.[lxiv] Some stroke

survivors have difficulty understanding emotions. The part of your

brain that is able to pick up on others facial expressions and their emotions may have been damaged by your stroke or brain injury.

Finding yourself struggling to process your emotions, and having difficulty picking up on subtleties of others' emotions is something that you can work on in speech therapy. Dr. John Miller, of the Stroke Recovery Association of British Columbia, explains that changes in mood are a common symptom for stroke survivors and recommends changing activities if you find yourself experiencing uncontrollable crying or laughing.

Resources

For individuals with aphasia suffering from depression, traditional talk therapy may not be an effective option. Seek out support groups, either on Facebook or in your community. The National Aphasia Association has a search page to help you find aphasia support groups near you. Visit: **aphasia.org/naa-network3**

Do not be embarrassed to seek out the help of a psychiatrist. You can bring a friend or family member with you to help express what you are feeling. You can also ask your speech therapist to help you write down your concerns before you meet with a psychiatrist. Remember, almost two thirds or people with aphasia are clinically depressed at the one year mark after their stroke.[lxv] It is very common for people with aphasia to have some depression. The key is to recognize it and take action.

Motivation

Try to push yourself to stay active and involved. If you are blessed with supportive people in your life, try not to let them do too much for you. Work hard to do the things you are able to do even if it takes longer. Carol shares, "I remember when David was young, he reminded me I should let him take the reigns.

I found it difficult to leave David alone for any length of time as he needed help for almost everything. After a rare outing, my husband and I returned home to find a basket of cookies on the kitchen table. Hmm, someone must have dropped by for a visit. I wondered who had come by while we were out. David's aphasia made it impossible to just ask him, *Who brought the cookies*? Although he would know the answer, his stroke left him unable to speak. We relied on yes-or-no questions or used gestures to communicate.

I began my usual questioning. *Was it Sue*? No, David shook his head, looking annoyed. I remembered that the speech therapist suggested starting with a broad question and then narrow it down.

Thinking of broader categories, I asked, *Was it a neighbor? Was it someone from church? Did someone from the office come by?* David nodded no, no, no as his brows furrowed. *David, I must write a thank you note. Let's take this slow.* He put his hand up, gesturing me to stop talking. *'I'*, he began again. *'I?'* *I can't think of anyone whose name starts with the letter 'i',* I said, feeling defeated.

Finally, as words failed him, David thought of another way to communicate. In exasperation, he opened the dishwasher. Inside, there were the tell tale signs that the cookies were made in my own kitchen. I smiled as I looked down at my son, the mystery baker. David, with his face beaming, repeated simply, *'I.'* *I indeed!* I said with a joy I hadn't felt in weeks.

I learned a valuable lesson that night. Had David asked me if he could bake cookies (which would have been asked with pantomime and gestures) while we were away, I would have said a very firm, *No.* Yet, there were many things David was capable of doing and it was important to focus on what he *could* do, not on what he couldn't. David proved that he could do things by himself and he didn't need my constant help. He wanted to surprise us and had even painstakingly lined the basket with a cloth napkin."

Hope

There is much to be hopeful for. Aphasia is not a terminal or progressive disease that gets worse over time. People continue to make progress even decades after their diagnosis. Just because your speech therapy benefits have ended for the year doesn't mean your recovery should. There are many resources available to you through support groups, Facebook, computer software, therapy apps, workbooks, and university clinics. In fact, sometimes there are so many options that it is overwhelming. Take time to educate yourself and day by day you will get through this.

You may have been told that aphasia rehabilitation only occurs in the first 6 months or year after your stroke or brain injury. Some therapists use the term *plateau* to describe when you've reached your maximum recovery potential. There is increasing evidence that recovery continues to occur years and even decades after the initial diagnosis of aphasia.[lxvi]

There is a growing consensus among Speech-Language Pathologists that a plateau in aphasia recovery does not exist. The spontaneous recovery period can last up to two years where someone with aphasia will make the most progress.[lxvii] People with aphasia can continue to make progress decades after their initial diagnosis as long as they continue to challenge themselves.

David is a good example of continued progress. He did not expect to see significant gains in year six. However, he participated in an intensive program where he received daily speech therapy, sometimes twice a day. He made amazing gains because he was challenging himself throughout the day. While his case may seem unusual, many ARC members have similar experiences.

If somebody tells you you have reached a plateau in therapy, ask what you can do differently in therapy to challenge yourself. Perhaps the exercises you were doing in therapy lacked variety and you need more real life situations to make further improvement. Ask to focus on different goals or use different techniques such as Melodic Intonation Therapy or incorporate technology into treatment.

Sometimes therapists use the term plateau because therapy benefits have ended although your potential for recovery has not. Perhaps your therapist does not specialize in aphasia therapy and your case requires someone with more experience with aphasia therapy.

That is not to say you don't have a good therapist. Many therapists specialize in various fields of speech therapy. ARC has found that whenever possible it is best to have a therapist who clearly specializes in aphasia therapy.

You have the ability to continue to make progress on your own. Speech therapy isn't magic and language recovery can happen throughout your day with continued effort on your part to challenge yourself. Speech-Language Pathologist Dr. Lori Bartels-Tobin explains, "Do not let anyone claim that stroke survivors cannot get better. Become empowered. Be insistent. It might take more time and effort, but it can be done. Get started now."[lxviii]

"Focus on what you can do. Not on what you cannot do."

- David Dow

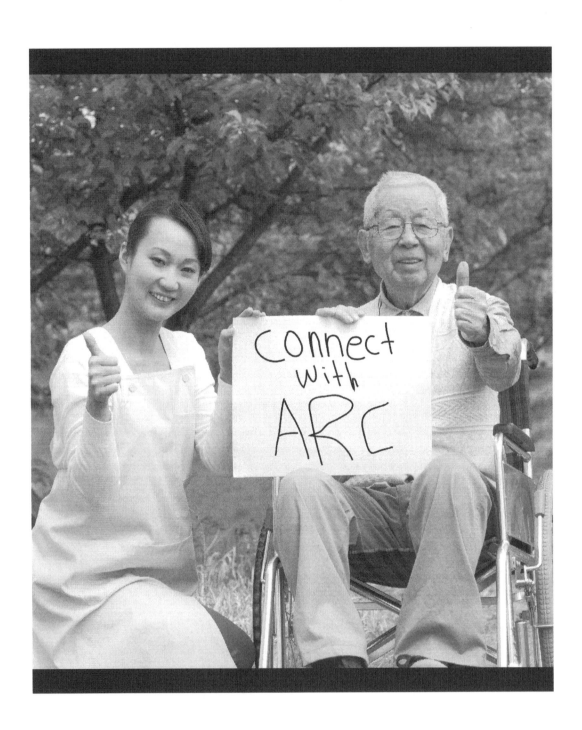

Chapter 9

Communication Strategies

ARC members have learned from experience how to improve communication using aphasia communication compensatory strategies. Make sure to try every mode of communication. If it works for you, then it's an excellent strategy! Writing, gestures, pointing, singing, reading, using picture cards, or communication technology are all viable options to improve communication.

Carol shares this account: "A few years ago, I was on a tour off a cruise ship. I noticed a man who appeared to be a stroke survivor. He had right-sided paralysis like my son David. I approached him, introduced myself, and asked him for his name. Silence, (as I thought might happen.) I proceeded to ask him if he could spell his name. Yes, he nodded. I opened the palm of my hand for him to draw the letter. Using his finger, he drew the letter J. *John? Jim? Jack?*, I asked. YES! His name was Jack.

Later, I saw Jack seated at dinner with his wife. I went to his table, introduced myself, and said, *Hi Jack. This must be your wife.* She glared at me. *How do you know my husband's name?*, she demanded. *He can't talk!* She seemed very angry. *I met Jack on the tour this morning. But he CANNOT TALK!* she insisted. *Perhaps not,* I said, *but he CAN communicate."*

Often, we think of aphasia recovery only about regaining speech. However, success in recovery also means finding new ways to communicate. It means adapting and finding new ways to find success in communicating like my friend Jack.

Sometimes seemingly obvious modes of communication can be missed by both Speech-Language Pathologists and caregivers. If there is something you can do that your family doesn't know about, try your best to let them know.

An ARC member shared her experience that emphasizes the importance of trying every mode of communication early on. She shares: "I didn't know for a year that my husband could read. One day my husband got agitated while I was on the computer. He hit the caps key and started banging the keyboard. It suddenly dawned on me that he wanted either to type or have me write in upper-case. I can't tell you what a new world it opened up to us. My husband now reads about ten pages a day. He is starting to understand lower-case and if he doesn't, I write it in upper-case for him."

Another ARC member shared this advice for people who have just been diagnosed with aphasia: "Be kind to yourself, you've been through a trauma. You might be tired, you might find that your emotions are out of control. Use any means you can to communicate: paper, pen, photos, gestures, whatever works for you. Rest if you can. Give yourself time."

Strategies for People with Aphasia

When meeting new people, it will be helpful to let them know you have aphasia. There are cards that you can purchase that explain that aphasia impacts language but not intelligence.

I Have Aphasia (From a Stroke):

This means I have difficulty with communication.
Please give me time to express myself.

Aphasia does NOT impact my intelligence

You can make your own card and personalize it with things that help improve your communication. The Aphasia Center's website has free pocket aphasia cards that you can customize and print out. Here is the link: **theaphasiacenter.com/pocket-card/**

Getting stuck on a particular word is one of the most common symptoms of aphasia. The key is to try your best not to get frustrated. Take a deep breath and think of other ways to say what you want. Don't get too focused on the specific word. There are other ways to get your point across. This moment is a perfect opportunity to build new neural pathways by using other modes of communication. Describing the word, gesturing, making sound effects, saying colors, location or writing the word are all options to communicate what you want to say.

When you get stuck on a particular word, it is useful to think of descriptive cues to communicate your point. Try to answer these questions:

Where do you find it?

What do you use it for?

When do you use it?

Who uses it?

Why do you use it?

How could you use it?

Show a gesture of yourself using it.

What sound does it make?

When you are stuck on a particular word, it is hard to take a deep breath and step back from focusing solely on the word itself and think of other ways you can express what you are trying to say.

Singing, drawing, writing, pointing, facial expressions and gestures are all great ways to express yourself. Use whatever works! One ARC member offers this advice: "Use as many senses as you can. Read out loud. Sing to the tune *Happy Birthday* as you read out loud. Bake cookies, read the newspaper out loud or have someone read the newspaper to you and discuss it. Look at family pictures and tell family stories. Put closed captioning on the TV. Make letters out of sandpaper and trace the words you make with the letters as you say them."

ARC members understand that communication can be exhausting. Determination to express yourself is key. Even if what you want to say is a small thing, every time you push yourself to communicate it is one step further in your rehabilitation. Don't be ashamed because it takes longer to express yourself.

Most people with aphasia experience well-meaning people who will attempt to finish your sentence for you. If this happens, try to say the word anyway and then say something like, "Thanks, but I can do it." Practice saying a phrase that will help you during conversations such as: "Just give me a minute.", "Give me a second, I can say it.", "I know it. I just need to find the word." You could put your hand up firmly, gesturing for them to stop. You need to take ownership and you will indeed have times where you want the other person to just stop guessing and simply give you time to try to get the word out.

To improve your comprehension, don't hesitate to ask somebody to repeat what they said. If writing down key points helps you, carry a whiteboard with you that says at the top, "please write that down". If you are able to understand what you read better than what you hear, you can use a whiteboard or a notepad app on a smartphone or tablet to have somebody write down what they said.

Adjusting to using your communication compensatory strategies will take time. It is essential that you learn to use them and not shy away from asking for accommodations because of pride or embarrassment. True friends will understand and be there for you, but it is important you give them the chance.

Communication Environment

The setting where you're trying to communicate can make a big difference on your ability to understand and express yourself. Try to limit distractions and background noise. Turn off the television and any background music. Make sure you can see the other person's face, which will help with comprehension. It is important to reduce background noise. Even small visual and auditory distractions can negatively impact communication.

David has tips to improve communication, "When you are speaking to somebody with aphasia, make sure you have their full attention before you start talking. When talking to people with aphasia, do not add unnecessary details. Emphasize key words. No two people with aphasia are exactly alike, but this is generally helpful for most of us."

Tips for Caregivers

It is essential that loved ones and key friends learn tips for aphasia. Communication is a two-way street. Carol recalls, "David and I were so frustrated in the beginning. I think we both cried every day for years." Aphasia is tough on you and your loved ones. Share this book with your loved ones to teach them how to best help you.

Carol shares, "Like many new caregivers, I was fumbling for solutions. Often, the TV was on as I didn't realize that the background noise was making it difficult for David while he was in the hospital. I would hover over David and constantly ask him yes-or-no questions. *Squeeze my hand for yes*, I'd say. *Do you want a blanket? Are you thirsty?* In fact, I developed a list of possibilities and would read it so I would not forget any possible issues he may want to communicate with me.

One particular afternoon, David was really frustrated. I'd read the entire list and he never squeezed my hand. Finally, I said, *Oh you want me to just be quiet?* David squeezed my hand so hard it hurt. So, with that, I leave you with the number one rule many people with aphasia want you to know: Sometimes they just want peace and quiet."

Helpful Tips for Your Caregiver

To improve comprehension for someone with aphasia, speak at a slow and steady pace. You do not need to speak louder unless they are hard of hearing. Before starting a conversation, set the topic and let them know what you are going to talk about. Repeat key points. Write down important points using a whiteboard or notepad. Use simple and clear gestures when you talk to help clarify your point. Try ᵎ

too much with your hands because it can be distracting. Eliminate

background noise.

Get in the habit of keeping a notepad or whiteboard with you so

you can write down key points. Notepads are helpful to write and draw

for both you and the person with aphasia. Try to keep your subject to

one topic at a time. Pause slightly between sentences and let them know

if the topic is going to change.

Don't pretend to understand when you really don't know what the

person with aphasia is trying to say. It isn't helpful to you or your loved

one to pretend what they said made sense. Recap after they speak to

make sure you understood correctly.

If a person with aphasia is having difficulty finding the right

word, do not finish their sentence for them. Instead, provide cues to

help them communicate their point. Ask if there is a gesture they can

use to explain what they mean. If they can write, ask them to write or

draw what they mean. Frustration is a natural aspect of anomia and

expressive aphasia. If the person with aphasia gets frustrated, you can

always come back to that thought in a few minutes and move on with

the conversation.

If you find yourself guessing what somebody with aphasia is trying to say, first try to make sure you are both talking about the same thing. Start with a broad category and then slowly narrow the subject down as you get information. Patience for both of you is important. If conversations get exhausting, try an activity that you can enjoy without having to talk. Some boardgames and card games require little language and would offer a nice break. Just because somebody has aphasia doesn't mean they want to be left alone.

It is important to know whether the person wants your help or not. If you think you know what they want to say, you might ask, "Would you like me to guess?" Give the person with aphasia the chance to ask for or deny assistance. All too often family members jump in, while the person with aphasia really wants to try to say it on their own and it is crucial for their recovery to allow them to try.

24-hour Therapy

Carol recalls the neurologist coming in and out of David's hospital room, saying very little. One day she ran after the doctor. Just as he was about to enter the elevator, she yelled, "Stop!" He looked stunned. Carol asked, "If this was your family member, what would you do?" The neurologist replied, "Stimulate, stimulate and challenge David to fight for his recovery. He has to try things, even if they are hard. That is the way to recovery."

Caregivers may be able to help improve language function at home. You do not have to be a speech therapist to help your loved one with aphasia with their recovery. The Life Participation Approach to aphasia supports the idea that family members can help optimize recovery during everyday communication and activities. Family members can play a huge role is recovery. ARC offers a subgroup for caregivers to provide feedback on ways you can help with language rehabilitation at home.

Speech therapy can focus on the interests of people with aphasia. If your family member with aphasia loves sports, animals or movies, make that the focus of conversation. Try to fill your activities with language throughout the day. You should not dwell on the mistakes, but instead focus on the positives. Do not criticize errors. After the person with aphasia says one or two words such as, "want up" model the correct sentence form and say "Okay, great. You want to get up."

Family members have the advantage of providing stimulation for language therapy in short intervals. Every time you speak together is an opportunity for improvement. Speech Therapy sessions can be long and exhausting especially for people with aphasia. Family members can stimulate speech all day long in short, manageable segments throughout the day. You can alternate between structured exercises and everyday conversation tasks.

The question, "What would you like for lunch?" can be expanded into an opportunity to target descriptive language. Have them describe to you the steps involved in making a sandwich or the ingredients that you will use when you make lunch. Have the person with aphasia read the directions from the cookbook for something that you are going to make, even if you have made it a thousand times and do not need to hear the directions. Enjoyable everyday language activities can be the best type of speech therapy.

Support

You and your family do not have to face aphasia alone. Aphasia Recovery Connection is a vibrant community of people with aphasia, caregivers and Speech-Language Pathologists eager to support you in your journey of recovery. ARC and its members are available to answer your questions online or offer many of the resources you need. ARC understands the unique journey that every individual with aphasia experiences and welcomes you with open arms. ARC "gets it," because they, too, have lived with the grief and challenges that aphasia has brought you and your loved ones. You are not alone on this journey. Join us!

Appendix A

Template to use in Hospital

Have your caregiver or family help you to complete the thoughts. This will help you communicate with the people around you.

— **I have aphasia.**

— **I worked as a _____.**

— **Aphasia does not affect my intellect.**

— **Please talk slowly.**

— **Emphasize key words so I can understand better.**

— **I can read. Write down key words.**

— **I communicate with _____**

— **My family members are: _____**

— **My hearing is fine. There is no need to yell.**

— **I am originally from: _____**

— **I _____ write.**

— **I love to_____.**

Appendix B

Contact Congress to repeal the Medicare Therapy Caps

Ask your legislators to show their support for repealing the therapy cap by cosponsoring H.R. 713/S. 367, the Medicare Access to Rehabilitation Services Act

Visit the following links to ask congress to repeal the Medicare Therapy Caps:

capwiz.com/asha2/issues/bills/?bill=62417966

capwiz.com/amerpta/issues/alert/?alertid=63223021&type=CO

Appendix C

How to join Facebook:

1. Open your web browser. Type in **facebook.com**

2. Under "Sign Up", type in your name, email address or mobile number, and create a password. You will use your email address or mobile number to log into Facebook.

3. Select your birthday, male or female, and then click the large green tab that says "sign up".

4. On the next page, you can follow the directions to "Find your friends" on Facebook or "skip this step" by clicking the option on the bottom of the box.

5. On the next two screens, you can "Fill out info" about yourself or skip the steps.

How to join Aphasia Recovery Connection's Facebook Group:

 Log in to Facebook. At the top of the page you will see a box that says "Find Friends". Type "Aphasia Recovery Connection" into this box. When the ARC page appears, click "Join Group" at the top of the page.

Appendix D

Quick Aphasia Resource Guide

<u>SUPPORT</u>

National Aphasia Association **www.aphasia.org**
National Stroke Association **www.stroke.org**
Brain Injury Association **wwwbiausa.org**
American Heart Association **www.strokeassociation.org**
ARC Facebook Group
www.facebook.com/groups/Aphasia.Recovery.Connection/
Phone Support: The WARMLINE by American Stroke Association:
1888-478-7653

<u>FAMILY SUPPORT AND EDUCATION</u>

ARC Caregiver Facebook site.
www.facebook.com/groups/146625638825426
Aphasia Simulations: **http://aphasiacorner.com/aphasia-simulations/**
What you need to know about Aphasia:
tactustherapy.com/5-ways-to-help-someone-with-aphasia/

<u>MAGAZINES / BOOKS FOR STROKE SURVIVORS</u>
Stroke Connection Magazine – Free from American Heart and Stroke
Association
http://www.strokeassociation.org/STROKEORG/StrokeConnectionMag
azine/InStroke-Connection-
Magazine_UCM_308575_SubHomePage.jsp
Stroke Smart Magazine – Free from National Stroke Association
http://www.stroke.org/site/PageServer?pagename=ma

BOOKS

Aphasia Recovery Connection's Guide to Living with Aphasia on Amazon Carol Dow-Richards and Amanda Anderson M.S. CCC-SLP

Brain Attack: My Journey of Recovery from Stroke & Aphasia on Amazon – David Dow

Speech Therapy Aphasia Rehabilitation *STAR* Workbooks I,II & III on Amazon
-Amanda Anderson M.S. CCC-SLP

APHASIA VIDEOS

Caregiver Video Tips with Dr. Audrey Holland:

https://www.youtube.com/watch?v=3rFWtWXMBtY

David Dow Story (Co-Founder of ARC who had a stroke at ten – includes communication tips)

http://www.youtube.com/watch?v=IHKUwBP0xNk

Sarah Scott Story (a young stroke survivor who shares her journey of recovery)

https://www.youtube.com/watch?v=rUTHNS45Qmc

Introduction to ARC: The Aphasia Recovery Connection

https://www.youtube.com/watch?v=FxpLvdEQxJA

LEARN MORE

National Aphasia Association Website
www.aphasia.org

Aphasia Recovery Connection Website
www.aphasiarecoveryconnection.org (ARC Website)

Aphasia Recovery Connection Public Page
https://www.facebook.com/aphasiaARC

OTHER APHASIA RECOVERY OPTIONS

ARC Aphasia University / Boot Camp: A 28 day intensive program with a 7-10 day "start up" in Las Vegas. Email ARCaphasia@gmail.com for more information or call Carol at 702-336-0200.

University Clinics: continued group and/or individual therapy
http://www.asha.org/students/edfind/browse/

A List of Intensive Aphasia Therapy Programs:
http://www.slandp.com/?p=56

ASHA Professional Locator: **http://www.asha.org/findpro/**

Academy of Neurologic Communication Disorders and Sciences:
http://ancds.org/index.php?option=com_comprofilerHYPERLINK "http://ancds.org/index.php?option=com_comprofiler&task=usersList&listid=7"&HYPERLINK "http://ancds.org/index.php?option=com_comprofiler&task=usersList&listid=7"task=usersListHYPERLINK "http://ancds.org/index.php?option=com_comprofiler&task=usersList&listid=7"&HYPERLINK "http://ancds.org/index.php?option=com_comprofiler&task=usersList&listid=7"listid=7

ARC Aphasia Cruises & Retreats: Join others sharing the same challenges and experiences at an ARC event. Email ARCaphasia@gmail.com for more information.

Glossary

AAC: Augmentative and Alternative Communication, typically a device that is used for communication.

ADLs: Activities of Daily Living, A term used in rehabilitation referring to routine activities that people tend to do everyday without needing assistance. There are six basic ADLs: eating, bathing, dressing, toileting, transferring (walking) and continence.

AFO: Ankle-foot orthosis: A brace, usually made of plastic that is worn on the lower leg and foot to support the ankle, hold the foot and ankle in the correct position and correct foot drop. Abbreviated AFO. Also known as foot drop brace.

ALF: Assisted Living Facility, residential community that provides nursing care, rehab services, and meals for residents.

Aneurysm: bulge or ballooning in a blood vessel.

Anomia: a form of aphasia in which the patient is unable to recall the names of everyday objects.

Aphasia: Aphasia is an impairment of language, affecting the production or comprehension of speech and the ability to read or write resulting from injury to the brain.

ASHA: American Speech-Language-Hearing Association (ASHA) is the national professional, scientific, and credentialing association for more than 173,070 members and affiliates who are audiologists; speech-language pathologists; speech, language, and hearing scientists; audiology and speech-language pathology support personnel; and students.

Aspiration Pneumonia: Pneumonia caused by food or liquid entering the airway and lungs as a result of dysphagia. Stroke survivors are at high risk for aspiration pneumonia which can be life threatening.

Brain Hemorrhage: Is a type of stroke caused by an artery in the brain bursting and causing localized bleeding in the surrounding tissues. This bleeding kills brain cells.

Brain Lesion: abnormal areas of tissue in in the brain.

Carotid Artery Dissection: is a separation of the layers of the artery wall supplying oxygen-bearing blood to the head and brain, and is the most common cause of stroke in young adults.

Circumlocutions: Talking around a word. Describing and using other words to explain what you are trying to say. This is actually a very positive technique and should be encouraged as a compensatory strategy.

CT Scan: A term for CAT scan which stands for computerized axial tomography scan. A CAT scan is a painless X-ray test where a computer takes cross-section views of your anatomy. Iodine contrast can be used to view the integrity of your artery walls and blood flow.

COTA: Certified Occupational Therapy Assistant. Requires an associate's degree.

Dysphagia: Difficulty swallowing.

Inpatient: Residential rehabilitation setting either in a hospital or skilled nursing facility.

Jargon: Fluent utterances that make little or no sense, often seen in receptive aphasia.[lxix]

MBS: Modified Barium Swallow. Procedure used to image the swallowing process. The patient consumes foods of varying consistencies that have been coated with barium to check for aspiration and risk of choking on a variety of liquid consistencies and food textures.

MRI: Magnetic resonance imaging is a technique that uses a magnetic field and radio waves to create detailed images of the brain to show location and size of injury.

M.S. CCC-SLP: Found after a speech therapists name. M.S stands for Master's Degree in Science, CCC stands for Certificate of Clinical Competence by the American Speech-Language-Hearing Association, and SLP stands for Speech-Language Pathologist.

Moyamoya Disease: is a rare hereditary condition in which certain arteries in the brain are constricted. Blood flow is blocked by the constriction, and also by blood clots.

NAA: National Aphasia Association (aphasia.org)

NPO: Nothing by mouth.

Oovoo: A free service that provides instant messaging, phone calling, video messages and video chatting with up to twelve other users.

OT: Occupational therapists: Occupational therapists apply their specific knowledge to enable people to engage in activities of daily living that have personal meaning and value. They focus on fine motor muscles and typically treat contractures and arm and hand muscle weakness for stroke survivors. Requires a Master's degree or clinical doctorate.

Outpatient: Non-residential rehabilitation setting in which you would receive therapy on an appointment basis.

Perseveration: The repetition of a particular response, such as a word, phrase, or gesture, despite the absence or cessation of a stimulus, usually a symptom of aphasia.

Phonemic Paraphasia: Substituting, adding or rearranging the speech sounds in a word.

PET SCAN: A positron emission tomography, A PET scan uses a radioactive drug (tracer) to show how your tissues and organs are functioning.

PM&R: Physical medicine and rehabilitation also called physiatry, is the branch of medicine emphasizing the prevention, diagnosis, and treatment of disorders that are particularly related to the nerves, muscles, and bones. These disorders that may produce temporary or permanent impairment.

PO: By mouth.

Power of Attorney: POA is a written authorization that gives someone permission to act legally on your behalf in financial, medical or legal matters.

Premorbid: before the symptoms of disease or disorder.

PT: Physical therapists, licensed health care professionals who can help patients reduce pain and improve or restore mobility. PTs evaluate and treat gross motor (large motor) muscle deficits and help stroke survivors with strengthening, transfers and mobility. Requires a Master's degree or clinical doctorate.

PTA: Physical therapist assistant. Requires an Associates degree.

Semantic Paraphasia: Substituting an incorrect word for another with or without recognizing the mistake.

Skype: a software application and online service that enables voice and video phone calls over the internet.

SLP: Speech-language pathologists identify, evaluate and treat speech and language problems, including swallowing disorders. Requires a Masters degree. Also referred to as Speech Therapists.

SNF: Skilled Nursing Facility, an inpatient facility that provides nursing care and rehabilitation services on either a short term or long term care basis.

Therapy Cap: Refers to Medicare Part B therapy cap presently allots $1,920 for Occupational Therapy and $1,920 for Physical and Speech Therapy services combined. Stroke survivors typically require both physical and speech therapy rehabilitation and the Medicare funds are rarely sufficient to provide full recover. To take action see Appendix B.

TBI: Traumatic Brain Injury is damage to the brain from an external mechanical force possibly leading to temporary or permanent impairment of cognitive and/or physical function.

Other Books By These Authors

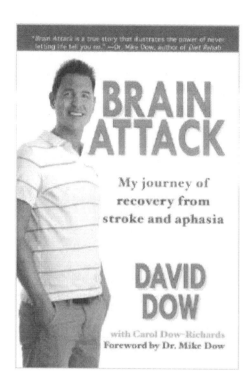

Brain Attack shares David's story with frankness, humor, and most of all, with hope. A great motivational read for people coping with aphasia.

To order: Search amazon.com for: "Brain Attack David Dow"

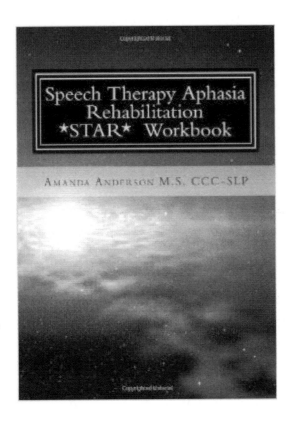

Speech Therapy Aphasia Rehabilitation *STAR* Workbooks

A series of three workbooks for people with aphasia to optimize recovery either in therapy or at home.

To order: Search Amazon: "Aphasia Workbook Anderson"

i American Heart Association. (2012) Lets Talk About Stroke and Aphasia, Retrieved from http://www.strokeassociation.org/idc/groups/heart-public/@wcm/@hcm/documents/downloadable/ucm_309703.pdf

ii National Institute for Neurological Disorders and Stroke (February 14, 2014). NINDS Aphasia Information Page. Retrieved from http://www.ninds.nih.gov/disorders/aphasia/aphasia.htm.

iii The American Heart Association (2014) Types of Strokes. Retrieved from http://www.strokeassociation.org/STROKEORG/AboutStroke/TypesofStroke/Types-of-Stroke_UCM_308531_SubHomePage.jsp

iv National Institute of Neurological Disorders and Stroke (2014) Ischemic Stroke. Retrieved from http://www.strokecenter.org/patients/about-stroke/ischemic-stroke/

v American Heart Association. (2014) Hemorrhagic Strokes (Bleeds). Retrieved from http://www.strokeassociation.org/STROKEORG/AboutStroke/TypesofStroke/HemorrhagicBleeds/Hemorrhagic-Strokes-Bleeds_UCM_310940_Article.jsp

vi National Heart Lung and Blood Institute. (2014) What is a Stroke? Retrieved from http://www.nhlbi.nih.gov/health/health-topics/topics/stroke/printall-index.html

vii American Heart Association. (2014) Hemorrhagic Strokes (Bleeds). Retrieved from http://www.strokeassociation.org/STROKEORG/AboutStroke/TypesofStroke/HemorrhagicBleeds/Hemorrhagic-Strokes-Bleeds_UCM_310940_Article.jsp

viii National Aphasia Association. (2011). Aphasia Facts. Retrieved from http://www.aphasia.org/content/aphasia-faq.

ix National Aphasia Association (2011) Aphasia FAQS. Retrieved from: http://www.aphasia.org/content/aphasia-faq

x National Aphasia Association (2011) Aphasia FAQS. Retrieved from: http://www.aphasia.org/content/aphasia-faq

xi Uwe Gille, CC-BY via: http://commons.wikimedia.org/wiki/Category:Broca%27s_area#mediaviewer/File:BrocasAreaSmall.png

xii Helm-Estabrooks, N, Albert, Martin L. (1991). Manual of Aphasia Therapy. Austin Texas: Pro-ed.

xiii Helm-Estabrooks, N, Albert, Martin L. (1991). Manual of Aphasia Therapy. Austin Texas: Pro-ed.

xiv UMN Communication Science department. Retrieved from: http://www.d.umn.edu/~mmizuko/2230/sym.htm

xv Lazar, M. R., Antoniello, D. (November, 2008). Variability in recovery from aphasia. Current Neurology and Neuroscience reports, 8(6). Retrieved from http://link.springer.com/article/10.1007/s11910-008-0079-x#page-1

xvi Helm-Estabrooks, N, Albert, Martin L. (1991). Manual of Aphasia Therapy. Austin Texas: Pro-ed.

xvii Lazar, M. R., Antoniello, D. (November, 2008). Variability in recovery from aphasia, Current Neurology and Neuroscience reports, 8(6). Retrieved from http://link.springer.com/article/10.1007/s11910-008-0079-x#page-1

xviii Lazar, M. R., Antoniello, D. (November, 2008). Variability in recovery from aphasia. Current Neurology and Neuroscience reports, 8(6). Retrieved from http://link.springer.com/article/10.1007/s11910-008-0079-x#page-1

xix National Stroke Association (August, 2012) Aphasia. Retrieved from http://www.stroke.org/site/PageServer?pagename=aphasia

xx National Aphasia Association. (2011). Aphasia Facts. Retrievedfrom http://www.aphasia.org/content/aphasia-faq.

xxi American Speech-Language-Hearing Association. (2014). Research Efficacy Summary. Retrieved from http://www.asha.org/uploadedFiles/public/speech/disorders/TESAphasiaFromLeftHemisphereStroke.pdf

xxii American Speech-Language-Hearing Association. (2014). Research Efficacy Summary. Retrieved from http://www.asha.org/uploadedFiles/public/speech/disorders/TESAphasiaFromLeftHemisphereStroke.pdf

xxiiiCenter For Disease Control and Prevention (2014). Cerebrovascular Disease or Stroke. Retrieved from http://www.cdc.gov/nchs/fastats/stroke.htm

xxivNational Stroke Association (2014) Rehabilitation Therapy After a Stroke. Retrieved from http://www.stroke.org/site/PageServer?pagename=REHABT

xxv American Stroke Association (March, 2013) Difficulty Swallowing After Stroke Dysphagia. Retrieved from http://www.strokeassociation.org/STROKEORG/LifeAfterStroke/RegainingIndependence/CommunicationChallenges/Difficulty-Swallowing-After-Stroke-Dysphagia_UCM_310084_Article.jsp.

xxviArcadian, CC-BY, Source: http://commons.wikimedia.org/wiki/File:Illu01_head_neck.jpg

xxviiUS News and World Report (2014) Top Ranked Hospitals for Rehabilitation. Retrieved from http://health.usnews.com/best-hospitals/rankings/rehabilitation

xxviiiASHA (2014) Telepractice Retrieved from http://www.asha.org/Practice-Portal/Professional-Issues/Telepractice/.

xxix Royal College of Speech Language Therapists (2011) Why do people lose friends after a stroke? Retrieved from: http://www.ncbi.nlm.nih.gov/pubmed/21899670

xxx Source: Uwe Gille, CC-BY, via: http://commons.wikimedia.org/wiki/File:BrocasAreaSmall.png

xxxi HOPES. (June 26, 2010). HOPES Huntington Outreach Project for Education at Stanford.

Retrieved from: http://www.stanford.edu/group/hopes/cgi-bin/wordpress/2010/06/neuroplasticity/

xxxiiPerlmutter, David MD,. (November 2, 2010). Neurogenesis: How to Change Your Brain. Retrieved from http://www.huffingtonpost.com/dr-david-perlmutter-md/neurogenesis-what-it-mean_b_777163.html

xxxiiiAmerican Stroke Association, (2014) retrieved from: http://powertoendstroke.org/stroke-reduce-risk-controllable.html.

xxxiv Ira S. Ockene I,S, MD, & Houston Miller, N. (November 11, 1997).Cigarette Smoking, Cardiovascular Disease, and Stroke A Statement for Healthcare Professionals From the American Heart Association Retrieved from http://circ.ahajournals.org/content/96/9/3243.full

xxxv Ira S. Ockene, I,S, MD, & Houston Miller, N. (November 11, 19997).Cigarette Smoking, Cardiovascular Disease, and Stroke A Statement for Healthcare Professionals From the American Heart Association Retrieved from http://circ.ahajournals.org/content/96/9/3243.full

xxxvi National Stroke Association, (2014) retrieved from: http://www.stroke.org/site/PageServer?pagename=STARS

xxxviiNational Stroke Association, (2014) retrieved from:
http://www.stroke.org/site/PageServer?pagename=STARS

xxxviiiNational Stroke Association (20114) retrieved from:
http://www.stroke.org/site/PageServer?pagename=symp.

xxxixGiroux, Holistic Brain Health better living for MS, Parkison's, Dystonia Stroke:
Neuroplasticity. retrieved from http://drgiroux.com/neuroplasticity/

xl Giroux, Holistic Brain Health better living for MS, Parkison's, Dystonia Stroke:
Neuroplasticity. retrieved from http://drgiroux.com/neuroplasticity/

xli Stroke Connection Magazine (September/October 2004)Constraint induced
movement therapy retrieved from
http://www.strokeassociation.org/STROKEORG/LifeAfterStroke/RegainingIndepen
dence/PhysicalChallenges/Constraint-Induced-Movement-
Therapy_UCM_309798_Article.jsp

xlii Friedemann Pulvermüller, PhD,Bettina Neininger, MA,Thomas Elbert, PhD, Bettina Mohr,
PhD, Brigitte Rockstroh, PhD. Peter Koebbel, MA, Edward Taub, PhD, (November 11,
2000). **Constraint-Induced Therapy of Chronic Aphasia After Stroke. Retrieved from
http://stroke.ahajournals.org/content/32/7/1621.full**

xliii Friedemann Pulvermüller, PhD,Bettina Neininger, MA,Thomas Elbert, PhD, Bettina Mohr,
PhD, Brigitte Rockstroh, PhD. Peter Koebbel, MA, Edward Taub, PhD, (November 11,
2000). **Constraint-Induced Therapy of Chronic Aphasia After Stroke. Retrieved from
http://stroke.ahajournals.org/content/32/7/1621.full**

xlivFriedemann Pulvermüller, PhD,Bettina Neininger, MA,Thomas Elbert, PhD, Bettina Mohr,
PhD, Brigitte Rockstroh, PhD. Peter Koebbel, MA, Edward Taub, PhD, (November 11,
2000). **Constraint-Induced Therapy of Chronic Aphasia After Stroke. Retrieved from
http://stroke.ahajournals.org/content/32/7/1621.full**

xlvASHA, (2014) Aphasia Treatments. Retrieved from
http://www.asha.org/PRPSpecificTopic.aspx?

xlvi Palmer, R., Enderby, P., et al. (2013). Using Computers to Enable Self-Management of
Aphasia Therapy Exercises for Word Finding: The Patient and Carer Perspective. Retrieved
from http://ncepmaps.org/aphasia/tx/comp-based/

xlviiHelm-Estabrooks, N, Albert, Martin L. (1991). Manual of Aphasia Therapy. Austin Texas:
Pro-ed.

xlviiiNorton, Andrea, Zipse,L, Schlaug, G. (2009) Melodic Intonation Therapy: Shared
Insights on How it is Done and Why it Might Help. Retrieved from:
http://www.ncbi.nlm.nih.gov/pmc/articles/PMC2780359/

xlixHelm-Estabrooks, N, Albert, Martin L. (1991). Manual of Aphasia Therapy. Austin Texas:
Pro-ed.

l Helm-Estabrooks, N, Albert, Martin L. (1991). Manual of Aphasia Therapy. Austin Texas:
Pro-ed.

li McCaffrey, Patrick. (2008) Neuroscience on the Web Aphasia Therapy. Retrieved
from http://www.csuchico.edu/~pmccaffrey/syllabi/SPPA336/336unit10.html

lii Cherney LR, (2010) Oral reading for language in aphasia (ORLA): evaluating the
efficacy of computer-delivered therapy in chronic nonfluent aphasia. Retrieved from
http://www.ncbi.nlm.nih.gov/pubmed/21239366

liii Holland, Audrey, (2011) Developing and Using Scripts in the Treatment of Aphasia. Retrieved from http://www.unm.edu/~atneel/shs531/aphasia-scripts2-handout.pdf

liv ASHA, (2014) Aphasia Treatments. Retrieved from http://www.asha.org/PRPSpecificTopic.aspx?folderid=8589934663&section=Treatment.

lv Sutton, M. (2012) App-titude: Apps to Aid Aphasia, ASHA LEADER Retrived from http://www.asha.org/Publications/leader/2012/120605/App-titude—Apps-to-Aid-Aphasia.htm.

lvi Kauhanen ML et al. (2000) Aphasia, depression, and non-verbal cognitive impairment in ischaemic stroke. Retrieved from: http://www.ncbi.nlm.nih.gov/pubmed/11070376

lvii Kauhanen ML et al. (2000) Aphasia, depression, and non-verbal cognitive impairment in ischaemic stroke. Retrieved from: http://www.ncbi.nlm.nih.gov/pubmed/11070376

lviii Jungfer, P, MD. (2014) Depression following Stroke. Retrieved from: http://www.strokensw.org.au/after-a-stroke/depression-following-stroke/

lix Jungfer, P, MD. (2014) Depression following Stroke. Retrieved from: http://www.strokensw.org.au/after-a-stroke/depression-following-stroke/

lx Benson, D. and Ardila, A. (1996) Aphasia a Clinical Perspective. Oxford University Press.. Retrieved from: http://books.google.com/books?id=iZ8PfkgGiOUC&pg=PA331&lpg=PA331&dq=aphasia+periods+of+grief&source=bl&ots=UB9h3vrAUm&sig=CpPqDY_hiuTlTp4UOgizzndfVIY&hl=en&sa=X&ei=eRzUU5zaB42yyATt0oL4Cg&ved=0CCgQ6AEwAg#v=onepage&q=aphasia%20periods%20of%20grief&f=false

lxi Friedman, R. (2009) No Stages of Grief Retrieved from: http://www.psychologytoday.com/blog/broken-hearts/200909/no-stages-grief

lxii Devine, M. (2013) Stages of Grief and Other Lies that don't help anyone. Retrieved From http://www.huffingtonpost.com/megan-devine/stages-of-grief_b_4414077.html

lxiii National Stroke Foundation (2014) Understanding Emotional Lability. Retrieved from: http://www.strokefoundation.com.au/blog/?tag=emotional-lability

lxiv National Stroke Foundation (2014) Understanding Emotional Lability. Retrieved from: http://www.strokefoundation.com.au/blog/?tag=emotional-lability

lxv Kauhanen ML et al. (2000) Aphasia, depression, and non-verbal cognitive impairment in ischaemic stroke. Retrieved from: http://www.ncbi.nlm.nih.gov/pubmed/11070376

lxvi National Aphasia Association, (2014) Aphasia Facts Retrieved from http://www.aphasia.org/content/aphasia-faq

lxvii Bartels-Tobin, Lori. (2010) Aphasia Survivors Take Charge of Their Own Recovery. Retrieved From: http://www.strokesmart.org/article?id=92.

lxviii Bartels-Tobin, Lori. (2010) Aphasia Survivors Take Charge of Their Own Recovery. Retrieved From: http://www.strokesmart.org/article?id=92.

lxix UMN Communication Science department. Retrieved from: http://www.d.umn.edu/~mmizuko/2230/sym.htm

Different language

Chat - cognitively -

Take days off.

Boundaries , & Safety measures

feel Guilt & do it anyway

Control

Healthy for me & for them

Made in the USA
Lexington, KY
12 February 2015